A PRIMER IN OPHTHALMOLOGY

A textbook for students

HAROLD A. STEIN, M.D., M.Sc (Ophth.), F.R.C.S. (C)

Professor of Ophthalmology, University of Toronto, Toronto, Canada
Chief, Department of Ophthalmology, Scarborough General Hospital, Scarborough, Ontario
Attending Ophthalmologist, Mt. Sinai Hospital, Toronto, Ontario
Past President, Contact Lens Association of Ophthalmologists, New Orleans, Louisiana
Past President, Canadian Ophthalmological Society, Ottawa, Canada
Past President, Joint Commission on Allied Health Personnel in Ophthalmology, St. Paul, Minnesota

BERNARD J. SLATT, M.D., F.R.C.S. (C)

Associated Professor of Ophthalmology, University of Toronto, Toronto, Ontario
Attending Ophthalmologist, Mt. Sinai Hospital, Toronto, Ontario
Attending Ophthalmologist, Scarborough General Hospital, Scarborough, Ontario

RAYMOND M. STEIN, M.D., F.R.C.S. (C)

Lecturer, University of Toronto, Toronto, Canada
Attending Ophthalmologist, Scarborough General Hospital, Scarborough, Ontario
Attending Ophthalmologist, Mt. Sinai Hospital, Toronto
Commissioner, Joint Commission on Allied Health Personnel in Ophthalmology, St. Paul, Minnesota

with 212 illustrations   34 in color

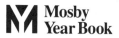
Mosby
Year Book

St. Louis   Baltimore   Boston   Chicago   London   Philadelphia   Sydney   Toronto

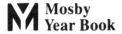

Mosby
Year Book
Dedicated to Publishing Excellence

Editor: Kimberly Kist
Assistant Editor: Penny Rudolph
Project Manager: John Rogers
Designer: Susan Lane
Cover Photo: © COMSTOCK, Inc.

Printed in the United States of America

Mosby–Year Book, Inc.
11830 Westline Industrial Drive
St. Louis, Missouri 63146

Library of Congress Cataloging in Publication Data

Stein, Harold A. (Harold Aaron), 1929–
    A primer in ophthalmology : a textbook for students / Harold A.
Stein, Bernard J. Slatt, Raymond M. Stein.
      p.   cm.
    Includes bibliographical references and index.
    ISBN 0-8016-4761-4
    1. Ophthalmology.   I. Slatt, Bernard J., 1934–   .   II. Stein,
Raymond M.   III. Title.
    [DNLM: 1. Eye Diseases.   WW 140 S819p]
RE46.S79   1992
617.7—dc20
DNLM/DLC
for Library of Congress

92 93 94 95 96   CL/CL/MV   9 8 7 6 5 4 3 2 1

TO OUR STUDENTS

who have encouraged us to help them understand
the fundamentals of eye disorders
and the acquisition of ophthalmic skills

Preface

This book is designed to bridge the gap of information between the exhaustive details found in some ophthalmic books to the minimal information provided in others. It is designed to fill the vacuum to provide essentials that are required to build a foundation in eye disorders.

The expanding technology in ophthalmology has created confusion in the minds of students as to how to differentiate important material from rarely needed information. Certainly, the explosion in ophthalmic lasers from Argon to Yag to Excimer has revolutionized our management of patients. The ever-changing techniques in cataract and implant surgery have restored sight to countless millions, but how much of these breakthroughs do students of medicine or optometry really need to know and remember? Tomorrow, these techniques will change, and new technology will come forward to arouse our interest.

Students are often faced with a three-part dilemma:

1. How can they learn quickly the skills that are required to perform good eye examinations?

2. How can they rule out disease processes of the eye and perhaps diagnose some of the common variations and some of the common pathological conditions?

3. When time is limited, which text should they purchase for a quick review of eye disorders and diseases? Existing textbooks are either extremely large and detailed and filled with concentrated facts or compact, too small, and omit much needed information.

We felt there was a need for a midway book that would be highly illustrated, that was neither heavy or burdensome to read, and that would provide practical instruction in developing ophthalmic skills.

This book was designed to be useful for students of medicine, optometry, beginning residents, and for family physicians who wish to quickly pick up the fundamentals of ophthalmic diagnosis. To this end, we hope we have achieved this goal.

We are indebted to many individuals for advice, but for the most part to our wives who have given up quality time for us to engage and produce this manuscript.

Harold A. Stein
Bernard J. Slatt
Raymond M. Stein

Contents

1 Basic anatomy and physiology of the eye

Although the eye is commonly called the *globe*, it is not really a true sphere. It is composed of two spheres with different radii, one set into the other (Figs. 1-1 and 1-2). The front, or anterior, sphere is the smaller and more curved of the two called the *cornea*. The cornea is the window of the eye, because it is a completely transparent structure. It is the more curved of the two spheres and sets into the other as a watch glass sets into the frame of a watch. The posterior sphere is a white opaque fibrous shell called the *sclera*. The cornea and the sclera are relatively nondistensible structures that encase the eye and form a protective covering for all the delicate structures within. The eye measures approximately 24 mm in all its main diameters in the normal adult.

SURFACE ANATOMY

The eye itself is covered externally by the eyelids, which are movable folds protecting the eye from injury and excessive light. The lids serve to swab the eye and spread a film of tears over the cornea, thereby preventing evaporation from the surface of the eye. The upper eyelid extends to the eyebrow, which separates it from the forehead, whereas the lower eyelid usually passes without any line of demarcation into the skin of the cheek. The upper eye is the more mobile of the two, and when the lid is open it covers about 1 mm of the cornea. A muscle that elevates the lid, the *levator palpebrae superioris*, is always active, keeping the eyelid open. During sleep the eyelid closes by relaxation of this muscle. The lower lid lies at the lower border of the cornea when the eye is open and rises slightly when it shuts.

Normally, when the eyes are open there is a triangular space visible on either side of the cornea. These triangular spaces, formed by the junction of the upper and lower lids, are called the *canthi* of the eye (Fig. 1-3). These canthi are denoted by the terms *medial* and *lateral*, medial being closer to the nasal bridge. Most eyes are practically the same size; therefore, when we speak of the eyes appearing large or small, we usually refer not to the actual size but to the portion of the eyeball visible on external exami-

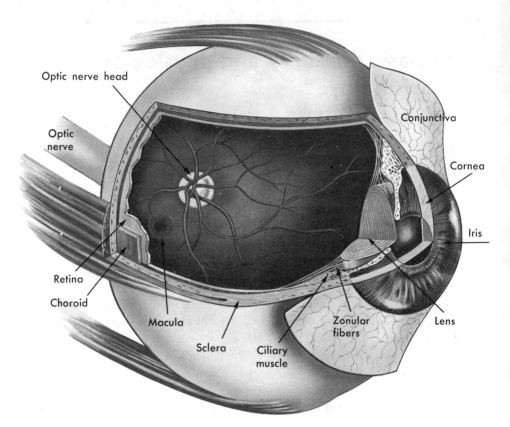

Optic nerve head

Optic nerve

Conjunctiva

Cornea

Iris

Retina

Choroid

Macula

Sclera

Ciliary muscle

Zonular fibers

Lens

Fig. 1-1 Cutaway section of the eye.

nation, which in turn depends on the size of the palpebral fissure. The shape of the fissure also determines its appearance. In Orientals, there is a fold of skin extending from the upper lid to the lower lid and covering the medial fissure, giving the eye its characteristic obliquity. In the medial fissure there are two fleshy mounds: the deeper one, called the *plica semilunaris*, and the superficial one, called the *caruncle* (Fig. 1-4). The caruncle is modified skin containing sweat and oil glands. Occasionally it also contains fine cilia, or hairs. When the eyes are open the palpebral fissures measure about 30 mm in width and 15 mm in height.

The free margin of each lid is about 2 mm broad and has an anterior and a posterior border. From the anterior, or front, border are the eyelashes, which are hairs arranged in two or three rows. The upper eyelid lashes are longer and more numerous than the lower, and they tend to curl upward. The lashes are longest and most curled in childhood. The posterior border of the lid margin is sharp and tightly abuts against the front surface of the globe. By depressing the lower lid, one can see a thin gray line that separates the two borders of the lid. This line, called the *gray line*, is used in many sur-

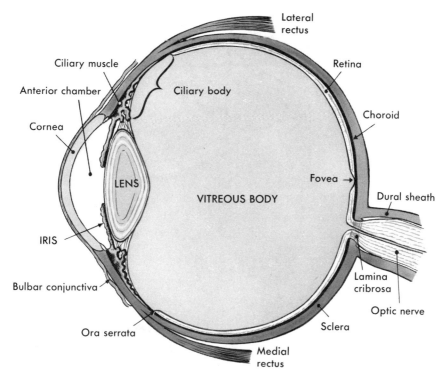

Fig. I-2 The eye cut in horizontal section.

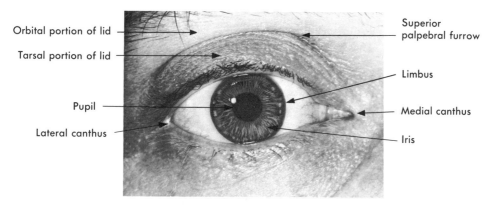

Fig. I-3 Surface anatomy of the eye.

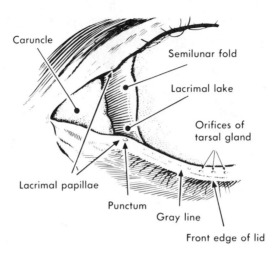

Fig. I-4   Inner canthus, showing the semilunar fold and the caruncle. Normally the punctum is not visible unless the lower lid is depressed.

gical procedures to split the upper and lower lids into two portions. Also visible on both lids are the tiny openings that are the orifices of the sweat- and oil-secreting glands. The largest oil-secreting glands are embedded in the posterior connective tissue substance of the lids (called the *tarsus*), and are called the *meibomian glands*. The lacrimal gland is located above and lateral to the globe. Tears are produced by the lacrimal gland and travel through fine channels called *ducts* to empty onto the conjunctival surface. On the medial aspect of the lower lid where the lashes cease is a small *papilla*. At the apex of this papilla is a tiny opening called the *punctum* (see Fig. 1-4). The punctum leads, by means of a small canal, through the lower lid to the *lacrimal sac* (Fig. 1-5), which eventually drains into the nose. Tears are carried to the punctum by the pumping action of the lids, and there they are drained effectively from the eye by means of tiny channels draining the punctum. A similar but smaller opening is found in the upper lid almost directly above it. The punctum normally cannot be seen by looking directly at the eye. It can be seen only by depressing the lower lid or everting the upper lid. The muscle underlying the eyelid skin is the *orbicularis oculi*, which is roughly circular. When it contracts it closes the eye.

The portions of the eye that are normally visible in the palpebral fissures are the cornea and sclera. Because the cornea is transparent, what is seen on looking at the cornea is the underlying *iris* and the black opening in the center of the iris, called the *pupil*. The sclera forms the white of the eye and is covered by a mucous membrane called the *conjunctiva*. The conjunctiva extends from the junction of the cornea and sclera and terminates at the inner portion of the lid margin (Fig. 1-6). The conjunctiva that covers the eye itself is called the *bulbar conjunctiva*, whereas the portion that lines the inner surface of the upper and lower lids is called the *palpebral portion*. The *junc-*

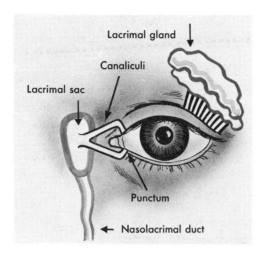

Fig. I-5   Lacrimal apparatus. Tears produced by the lacrimal gland are drained through the punctum, lacrimal sac, and nasolacrimal duct into the nose.

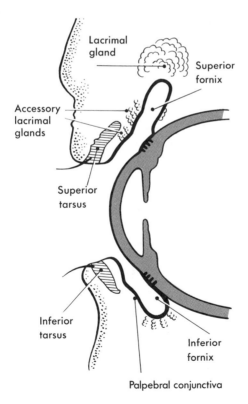

Fig. I-6   Vertical section of the eyelids and conjunctiva. The lids act as a protective curtain for the eye. Only a small portion of the eye is actually exposed.

tional bay created when the two portions of the conjunctiva meet is called the *fornix.* The lower fornix can easily be viewed by depressing the lower lid.

CORNEA

The cornea is a clear, transparent structure, with a brilliant, shiny surface. It has a convex surface that acts as a powerful lens. Most of the refraction of the eye takes place not through the crystalline lens of the eye but through the cornea.

The cornea is relatively large at birth and attains almost its adult size during the first and second years. Although the eyeball as a whole increases a little less than three times in volume from birth to maturity, the corneal segment plays a small role in this part, being fully developed by 2 years of age.

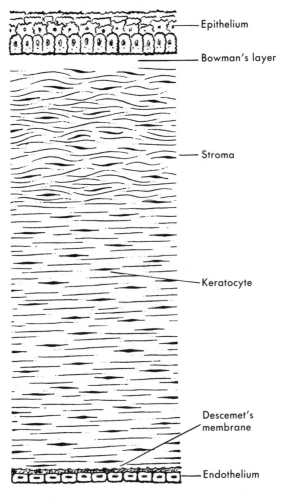

Fig. 1-7   The five layers of the cornea.

The cornea is thicker at its periphery (1 mm) than at the center (0.5 mm).
The cornea may be separated into five layers (Fig. 1-7):
- Epithelium (and its basement membrane)
- Bowman's layer
- Stroma
- Descemet's membrane
- Endothelium

Corneal epithelium

Functions. The major functions of the corneal epithelium are:
- Providing a mechanical barrier to microorganisms and foreign matter
- Maintaining a barrier to the diffusion of water and solutes
- Creating a smooth, transparent optical surface to which the tear film can adsorb

Structure. The epithelium consists of five to seven cell layers with three cell types:
basal cells, wing cells, and superficial flattened cells (Fig. 1-8). The basal cells are the
deepest layer and comprise a single layer of columnar cells that rest on the basement
membrane. These cells are connected to the underlying basement membrane by
hemidesmosomes. These focal spots extend through the basement membrane to Bowman's layer. Any clinician who has attempted to remove a normal corneal epithelium
with a moistened Q-tip or a scalpel blade appreciates the tenacity of the adhesion. The

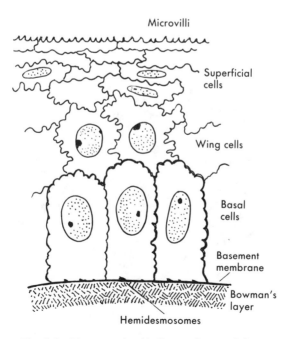

Microvilli

Superficial
cells

Wing cells

Basal
cells

Basement
membrane

Bowman's
layer

Hemidesmosomes

Fig. I-8   The corneal epithelium to Bowman's layer.

wing cells, of which there are two layers, and the superficial flattened cells, of which there are three layers, complete the epithelium. The multisided wing cells interlock with each other and adhere with large numbers of desmosomal attachments to the adjacent cell. These desmosomal attachments consist of tonofilaments that extend across the intercellular space from the plasma membrane of one cell to an adjacent cell. The most superifical cells are flat, overlapping squamous cells, similar to the most superfical epithelial cells of the skin. Normal corneal epithelium is not keratinized. The surface epithelial cells are uniform and smooth and have desmosomal intercellular attachments. In addition these surface cells are zippered together by *zonulae occludentes* (tight junctions), which encircle the cells and consist of adhesion of the two adjacent plasma membranes. This strong barrier blocks the penetration of most microorganisms and prevents the flow of fluid and electrolytes from the tears to the stroma, which assists in keeping the corneal stroma in a state of relative dehydration.

By electron microscopy the outer cell membranes of epithelial cells show fingerlike projections known as *microvilli* (Fig. 1-9). These microvilli project into the tear film and may trap tear fluid and thus prevent drying of the epithelial cells. There is a continuous migration of epithelial cells from the basal surface toward the tear film. Dividing basal cells become the wing-shaped cells that migrate superficially as flattened squamous cells and ultimately lose their attachments to the cornea and slough into the tear film. The corneal epithelium replaces itself about once a week.

Fluid can accumulate in the epithelium both intracellularly and extracellularly. Intracellular fluid expands the cells into round vesicles. The extracellular fluid accumu-

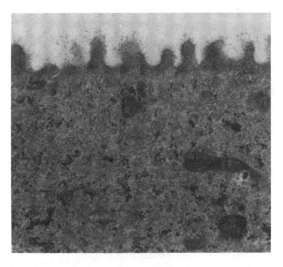

Fig. 1-9   Microvilli of the surface of the cornea; magnification × 36,600; (Courtesy Dr. Adolph I Cohen; from Moses RA and Hart WM: *Adler's physiology of the eye*, ed 8, St Louis, 1987, The CV Mosby Co.)

lates between the cells, which continue to remain attached by desmosomes. These pockets of fluid produce a microcystic texture, which is easily appreciated with a slit-lamp, and act to diffract light, which creates the halos that are described by patients with epithelial edema.

The basal cells of the epithelium are attached to the underlying basement membrane. If the basement membrane is damaged it can be regenerated by the epithelium. Abnormalities of the basement membrane appear most commonly in disorders such as recurrent corneal erosion, epithelial basement membrane dystrophy, and diabetes mellitus. Abnormal adhesion of the epithelium and abnormal secretion of basement membrane frequently result in surface irregularity with blurred vision and occasional painful erosions.

Bowman's layer and stroma

Functions. These layers perform three functions:
- They are transparent, so they allow the transmission of light.
- They maintain a fixed shape so that the cornea can function optically.
- They protect the intraocular contents.

Bowman's layer

On the posterior side of the epithelial basement membrane lies Bowman's layer. By light microscopy this layer is seen as a relatively homogeneous, acellular sheet and in the past was called *Bowman's membrane*. However, as seen by electron microscopy, this zone is a specialized layer resembling corneal stroma and is not a true membrane. It is a condensation of the superficial stroma, which consists of collagen fibrils. The layer cannot be detached from the stroma into which it imperceptibly blends. Unlike the epithelial basement membrane or Descemet's membrane, it cannot be replaced, and so, following injury, it may become opacified by scar tissue. There are tiny perforations in Bowman's layer that permit passage of corneal nerves to the epithelium.

Stroma

The stroma, which constitutes about 90% of the corneal thickness, consists primarily of collagen fibers, a ground substance, and keratocytes. The collagen fibers of the corneal stroma are uniform and small, about 250 to 300 Å (Fig. 1-10). Bundles of collagen fibers constitute lamellae, which stretch from limbus to limbus. The collagen bundles in the anterior zone are small and are neither as clearly defined nor as regular in size and arrangement as those found in the posterior portion of the stroma. Lamellae cross each other at right angles in a regular fashion, and layers of lamellae run parallel to each other and to the surface of the cornea. The ground substance consists of keratin sulfate and chondroitin sulfate and fills all the space not occupied by the fibrils and cells in the corneal stroma. In swollen corneas the volume of the ground substance increases, but the individual collagen fiber size does not change. The stroma also consists of keratocytes, which lie between the corneal lamellae and are capable of synthesizing collagen

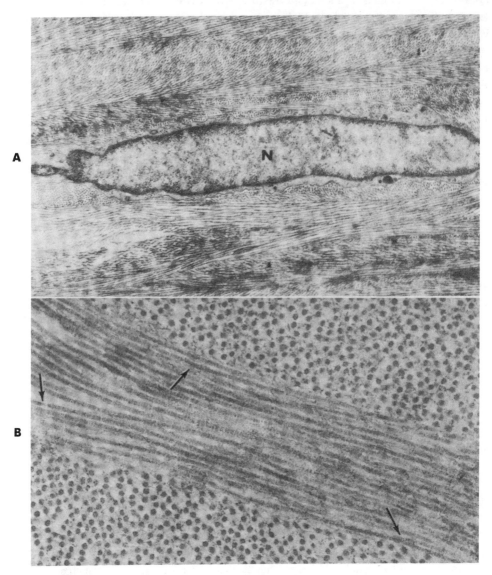

Fig. 1-10   A, Electron micrograph showing the nucleus, N, of a keratocyte and layers of corneal stromal collagen are seen from various angles; magnification ×9000. **B,** Higher magnification of stromal collagen, showing collagen fibrils cut on end and visible from side *(arrows)*; magnification ×72,000; (Courtesy Dr Jack Kayes; from Moses RA and Hart WM: *Adler's physiology of the eye,* ed 8, St Louis, 1987, The CV Mosby Co.)

and mucoprotein. Other freely moving cells seen in the stroma include histiocytes, lymphocytes, and, occasionally, polymorphonuclear leukocytes. These cells are generally present in response to some abnormal condition, and there is some disagreement as to whether they can be seen in a normal healthy cornea.

Descemet's membrane

Descemet's membrane is produced by the endothelium. Its thickness increases with age. At birth it is approximately 3 to 4 μ; in adulthood it is approximately 10 to 12 μ. The anterior portion of the membrane, which is adherent to the stroma, is fibrous and banded, while the posterior portion, adjacent to the endothelial cells, is a more homogeneous, nonbanded granular material (Fig. 1-11). The anterior portion of Descemet's membrane is the "oldest" portion and therefore the earliest to be laid down during fetal life. In contrast, the posterior portion is the youngest portion of the membrane and the part in which new material is continuously being laid down.

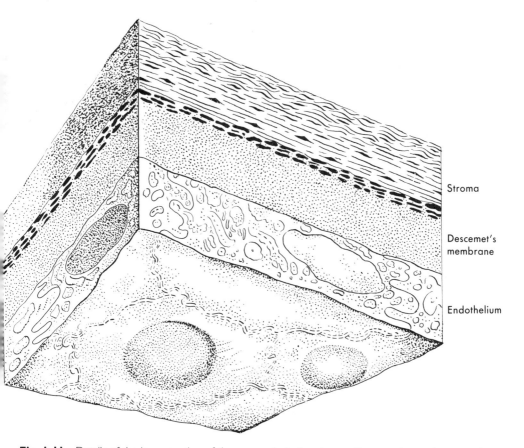

Stroma

Descemet's membrane

Endothelium

Fig. 1-11 Details of the inner portion of the cornea, including stroma, Descemet's membrane, and endothelium.

In contrast to Bowman's layer, Descemet's membrane is easily detached from the stroma, and it regenerates readily after injury. Excrescences or thickenings of Descemet's membrane may occur as a normal aging change in the peripheral cornea and are known as *Hassall-Henle warts*. These are considered abnormal when they occur in the central cornea (corneal guttata).

Endothelium

Functions. The corneal endothelium has a number of important functions. It functions as:

- A permeability barrier, allowing the diffusion of nutrients to the cornea
- A pump mechanism to maintain the cornea in a partially dehydrated state

Structure. Lining the posterior surface of the cornea and forming the anterior boundary of the anterior aqueous chamber is a single layer of cells known as the corneal endothelium. The endothelial cells are flat and hexagonal and are in direct contact with the aqueous humor. This cell layer has limited, if any, reproductive capacity. The endothelial surface can be visualized and photographed in vivo with the clinical specular microscope.

Aging causes endothelial cell loss, and the remaining cells enlarge, reorganize, and migrate to maintain the intact monolayer so that Descemet's membrane remains completely covered. Therefore, endothelial cell density, expressed as cells per unit area, decreases with age. Similarly, cell loss from trauma, inflammation, or intraocular surgery is compensated for by increased cell size and decreased cell density. Although some cells enlarge in response to aging or disease, other cells remain the same size, so the original homogeneous endothelial population gradually becomes heterogeneous. The cell density at birth is approximately 3000 cells per mm^2 and generally decreases with age. However, one cannot look at an endothelial photograph and accurately predict an individual's age, because there is often significant variation in cell density within various age-groups.

The functional capacity of the endothelium does not correlate well with cell density. As the cells enlarge, they can maintain a functional capacity that keeps the cornea clear. However, as the cell density drops below 500 cells per mm^2, the functional reserve is minimal and corneal edema is likely to appear.

Maintenance of corneal transparency

The corneal stroma has a natural tendency to imbibe water because of two forces:

- The intraocular pressure pushes the aqueous humor into the stroma.
- The glycosaminoglycans exert an osmotic pressure called the swelling pressure that pulls water into the stroma. Corneal transparency is maintained by the endothelium by counteracting this hydrophilic tendency by a pump function, which transports water out of the stroma, and by a barrier function, which decreases the flow of water into the stroma (Fig. 1-12).

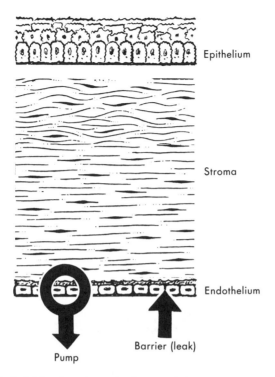

Fig. 1-12 Two endothelial functions that maintain corneal deturgescence: the leaky barrier and the metabolic pump. (Modified from Waring GO, Bourne WM, Edelhauser HF, and Kenyon KR: The corneal endothelium: normal and pathologic structure and function, Ophthalmology 89:531, 1982.)

The endothelial barrier is normally leaky to water; however, the leak rate normally equals the ability of the endothelium to pump water back out of the stroma. The stromal water content remains relatively constant at about 78% by weight and the corneal thickness remains relatively constant at approximately 0.56 mm.

The endothelial cells are attached to each other by a variety of junctions that do not form a tight barrier to the passage of small molecules and water, unlike the zonulae occludentes of the surface epithelial cells. This allows nutrients to freely penetrate the posterior layer of the cornea. The endothelial pump, an energy-dependent mechanism, results in ions being transported from the stroma to the aqueous humor, creating an osmotic gradient that draws water out of the stroma. This allows the stroma to maintain a partially dehydrated state that is necessary for the transmission of light to occur.

Corneal nerves

The cornea is richly supplied with sensory nerves. From 12 to 16 large, radially oriented nerve branches enter the cornea at the midstromal level at various clock positions

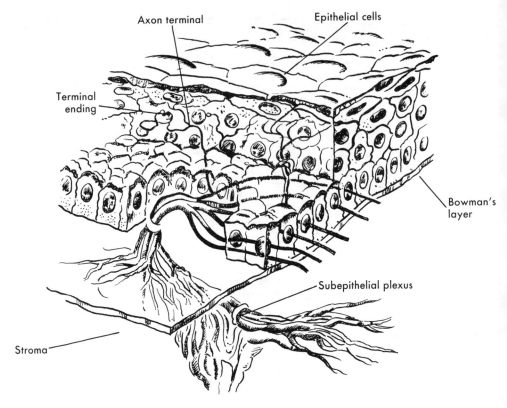

Fig. 1-13   Corneal nerves travel through the stroma, pierce Bowman's layer, and then supply sensation to the epithelium. (Modified from Rozsa AJ and Beuerman RW: Density and organization of free nerve endings in the corneal epithelium of the rabbit, Pain 14:105-120, 1981.)

around the limbus. The nerves travel in a radial fashion toward the center of the cornea; they branch horizontally and vertically, forming a dense subepithelial plexus beneath Bowman's layer. From this plexus, axonal extensions pass through Bowman's layer and into the epithelium to provide sensation (Fig. 1-13).

The nerve fibers generally lose their myelin sheaths when they have traversed 1 to 2 mm from the limbus; thus in the periphery of the cornea they often can be seen as fairly thick fibrils.

The cornea is one of the most sensitive tissues of the body, and this sensitivity serves to protect it. It can be exquisitely painful when the nerve endings are exposed, as in corneal abrasions or ulcers.

SCLERA

The opaque sclera forms the posterior five sixths of the protective coat of the eye. Its anterior portion is visible and constitutes the white of the eye. In children the sclera is thin, and therefore it appears bluish because the underlying pigmented structures are visible through it. In old age it may become yellowish because of the deposition of fat. Attached to the sclera are all the extraocular muscles. Through the sclera pass the nerves and the blood vessels that penetrate into the interior of the eye. At its most posterior portion, the site of attachment of the *optic nerve,* the sclera becomes a thin, sieve-like structure called the *lamina cribrosa.* It is through this sieve that the retinal fibers leave the eye to form the optic nerve. The episcleral tissue is a loose connective and elastic tissue that covers the sclera and unites it with the conjunctiva above. Unlike the sclera, the episcleral tissue is highly vascular.

UVEA

The uveal tract consists of three structures: *iris, ciliary body,* and *choroid.*

Iris

The iris is the most anterior structure of the uveal tract. It is perforated at its center by a circular aperture called the *pupil.* The surface of the iris has many ridges and furrows on its anterior surface. Contraction of the iris, which occurs in response to bright light, is accomplished by the activity of a flat, washerlike muscle buried in its substance just surrounding the pupillary opening. This muscle is called the *sphincter pupillae.* Expansion or dilation of the pupil is facilitated by relaxation of the sphincter muscle and by activation of the dilator muscle of the iris found at its peripheral circumference. Expansion and contraction of the iris, like an accordion, form circular pleat lines or furrows visible on its surface. In addition to these ridges and furrows on the surface of the iris, numerous white zigzag lines are formed by the blood vessels of the iris. Between the iris and the cornea is a clear fluid called the *aqueous humor.* This fluid occupies the space called the *anterior chamber* of the eye.

Ciliary body

The ciliary body is in direct continuity with the iris and is adherent to the sclera. Directly posterior to the iris, the ciliary body is plump and thrown into numerous folds referred to as the *ciliary processes.* This portion of the ciliary body is only about 2.5 mm in length and is responsible for the major production of aqueous fluid. The equator of the lens is only 0.5 mm from the ciliary processes and is suspended by fine, ligamentous fibers known as the *zonular fibers* of the lens. The posterior portion of the ciliary body is flat. Most of the zonular fibers of the lens originate from the ciliary body. The ciliary body in general is triangular, with its shortest side anterior. The anterior side of the triangle in its inner part enters into the formation of the angle of the anterior chamber. From its middle portion the iris takes root.

On the outer side of the triangle is the ciliary muscle, which lies against the sclera. Contraction of the ciliary muscle releases the tension of the zonular fibers, controlling the size and shape of the lens. This in turn allows the anterior surface of the lens to bulge forward and increase its power. Therefore, the ciliary muscle directly controls the focusing ability of the eye. In children this muscle is extremely active, and the lens is easily deformed, which accounts for their powerful ranges of accommodation, or focusing abilities. The ciliary muscle declines in power with age. After the age of 40 years, its power becomes weaker, and the lens is less able to change shape, so that focusing at near, or accommodating, becomes difficult. This condition is commonly called *presbyopia.*

Choroid

The choroid is in direct continuity with the iris and ciliary body and lies between the retina and sclera (see Fig. 1-2). The choroid is primarily a vascular structure, and its prime function is to provide nourishment for the outer layers of the retina.

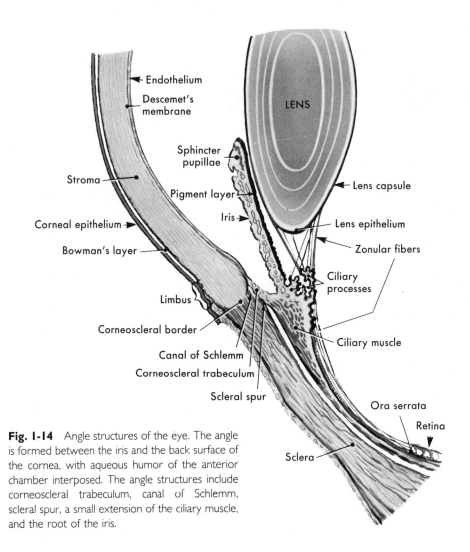

Fig. 1-14 Angle structures of the eye. The angle is formed between the iris and the back surface of the cornea, with aqueous humor of the anterior chamber interposed. The angle structures include corneoscleral trabeculum, canal of Schlemm, scleral spur, a small extension of the ciliary muscle, and the root of the iris.

ANGLE STRUCTURES

The angle structures are formed by the tissues posterior to the cornea and anterior to the iris, the aqueous humor intervening (Fig. 1-14). Included in the angle structures are (1) the root of the iris, (2) a portion of the anterior surface of the ciliary body, (3) a spur from the sclera, (4) the canal of Schlemm, and (5) the corneoscleral trabeculum.

Aqueous humor leaves the eye by filtering through the crevices of the trabecular meshwork. The trabecular meshwork has tiny pores through which aqueous humor travels until it reaches the canal of Schlemm. From the canal of Schlemm the aqueous humor leaves the eye through the aqueous veins penetrating the sclera. Obstruction within the trabecular meshwork or the angle structures, by iris or scar tissue, results in glaucoma.

LENS

The lens of the eye is a transparent biconvex structure situated between the iris and the vitreous (Fig. 1-15). Only that portion of the lens not covered by iris tissue (that is, only that portion directly behind the pupillary space) is visible. The center of the anterior surface of the lens, known as its *anterior pole*, is only about 3 mm from the back surface of the cornea. The diameter of the lens is about 9 to 10 mm. Its peripheral margin, called the *equator*, lies about 0.5 mm from the ciliary processes. It is attached to the ciliary processes and to the posterior portion of the ciliary body by means of fine suspensory ligaments referred to as the *zonular fibers* (Fig. 1-16).

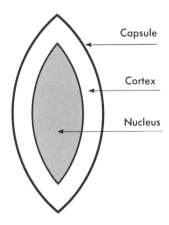

Fig. 1-15   Crystalline lens.

Capsule

Cortex

Nucleus

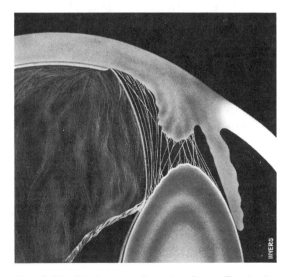

Fig. 1-16   Distribution of zonular fibers. Zonular lamella forms external layer of lens capsule consisting of anterior insertion 1 mm from equator and posterior insertion 1.5 mm from equator. (From Jaffe NS: *The vitreous in clinical ophthalmology,* St Louis, 1969, The CV Mosby Co.)

The lens is surrounded by a capsule, which is a transparent, highly elastic envelope. The lens material within this elastic bag is rather soft and puttylike in infants. With age it tends to grow harder, especially toward the center of the lens. The harder central portion of the lens found in adults 30 years of age or older is called the *nucleus* of the lens, and the outer lens fibers form the lens cortex. The harder nucleus is a product of the normal developmental growth of the lens. As new lens fibers are produced, the older fibers are pushed more toward the center and are compressed in a concentric fashion. It is this constant lamination of lens fibers over a period of years that eventually produces the nucleus of the lens.

VITREOUS

The vitreous is a jellylike structure, thick and viscous, that occupies the vitreous chamber in the posterior concavity of the globe. Actually, it fills the largest cavity of the eye, occupying two thirds of its volume. It is surrounded in the main by retina. Anteriorly it forms a slight depression behind the lens and is attached to it around the circumference of this depression. Normally the vitreous is quite transparent.

RETINA

The retina, which contains all the sensory receptors for the transmission of light, is really part of the brain. The retinal receptors are divided into two main populations— the *rods* and the *cones.* The rods function best in dim light; the cones function best under daylight conditions. The cones are far fewer in number than the rods, numbering 6 million, whereas the rods number 125 million. Cones enable us to see small visual angles with great acuity. Vision with rods is relatively poor. Color vision is totally dependent on the integrity of the cones. The cones form a concentrated area in the retina known as the *fovea,* which lies in the center of the *macula lutea.* Damage to this area can severely reduce the ability to see directly ahead. The rods are distributed in the periphery of the retina (not in the macula). Damage to these structures results in night blindness but with retention of good visual acuity for straight-ahead objects.

The junction of the periphery of the retina and the ciliary body is called the *ora serrata.* In the extreme periphery of the retina there are no cones and only a few rods. The retina is firmly attached to the choroid at the ora serrata. This is the reason that retinal detachments never extend beyond the ora serrata. The other site of firm attachment of the retina is at the circumference of the optic nerve. The posterior layer of the retina, called the *pigment epithelium,* is firmly secured to the choroid. Retinal detachment occurs as a result of cleavage between its anterior layers and the posterior pigment layer.

OPTIC NERVE

The optic nerve is located at the posterior portion of the globe and transmits visual impulses from the retina to the brain itself. Only the head of the optic nerve, called the *optic disc,* can be seen by ophthalmoscopic examination (Fig. 1-17). The optic nerve

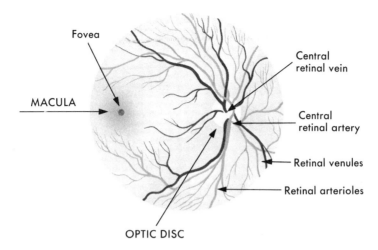

Fig. 1-17   Normal fundus. Note that the central retinal vein emerges from the optic disc lateral to the central retinal artery.

contains no sensory receptors itself, and therefore its position corresponds to the normal blind spot of the eye. Branching out from the surface of the optic disc are the *retinal arterioles* and *veins*, which divide soon after leaving the optic disc and extend out on the surface of the retina to supply the inner one third with nutriments. As the optic disc enters the globe, it goes through a fibrous, sievelike structure, visible on ophthalmoscopic examination, called the *lamina cribrosa*. When the lamina cribrosa is prominent, it forms the base of a depression in the disc called the *physiologic cup*. The optic nerve consists of 1 million axons arising from the ganglion cells of the retina. The nerve emerges from the back of the eye through a small circular opening; it extends for 25 to 30 mm and travels within the muscle cone to enter the bony optic foramen, where it travels for 4 to 9 mm to pass into the intracranial cavity and joins its fellow optic nerve to form the optic chiasm.

VISUAL PATHWAY

As the retinal fibers leave the optic nerves, half of them cross to the opposite side (Fig. 1-18). The fibers that cross are derived from the retinal receptors nasal to the macula. The structure so formed by the mutual crossing of nasal fibers by both optic nerves is the *optic chiasm*. From the optic chiasm the nasal fibers emanating from the nasal half of the retina of one eye intermingle with the fibers derived from the temporal sector of the retina of the opposite eye, forming a band called the *optic tract*. Fibers in the optic tract continue toward a cell station in the brain called the *lateral geniculate body*, so named because this body in the brain is shaped like a knee (Latin *genu*). The geniculate body is a relay station. From here, fibers spread out in a fan-shaped manner and extend to the parietal and temporal lobe of the brain. They continue to their final destination,

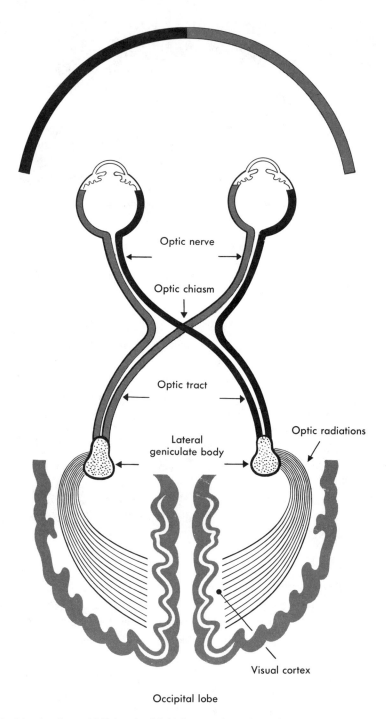

Optic nerve

Optic chiasm

Optic tract

Optic radiations

Lateral
geniculate body

Visual cortex

Occipital lobe

Fig. 1-18 Visual pathway. Half the visual field from each eye is projected to one side of the brain. Thus visual impulses from the right side of the retina of each eye will be transmitted to the left occipital lobe.

the posterior portion of the brain called the *occipital lobe* in an area denoted as the *visual striate area.* It is in this area of the brain that conscious recognition of visual impulses takes place.

OCULAR MUSCLES

The globe is moved by six ocular muscles: the *medial, lateral, superior,* and *inferior rectus muscles,* and the *superior* and *inferior oblique muscles* (Fig. 1-19). The medial rectus muscle moves the eye toward the nose, or *adducts* the eye. The lateral rectus muscle moves the eye horizontally to the outer side, or *abducts* the eye. The superior rectus muscle elevates the eye primarily, whereas the inferior rectus muscle depresses the eye. The recti muscles are inserted very close to the limbus, the medial rectus lying approximately 5.5 mm and the lateral rectus approximately 7 mm from the limbus. The rectus muscles normally are not visible, because they are covered with conjunctiva and subconjunctival tissue. Because they lie on the surface of the globe they are readily accessible for muscle surgery. The superior oblique muscle functions primarily as an intorter (turns the eye on its axis inward) by rotating the vertical and horizontal axis of the eye toward the nose; it also functions to depress the eye. The inferior oblique muscle acts to extort the eye (to turn the eye outward) and also serves to elevate the eye. The oblique muscles are inserted behind the equator of the globe.

In the lid the *levator palpebrae superioris muscle* serves to elevate the lid, whereas the *orbicularis oculi muscle* closes the eye during winking, blinking, or forced lid closure. If the levator muscle is weak or absent, the lid droops and ptosis results.

SUMMARY

Each of the structures of the eye, when diseased, gives rise to problems, depending on their anatomic location and function. Since many diagnoses made in ophthalmology are formulated from anatomic terminology, familiarity with these structures is essential before any understanding of patients' problems can be realized. The foundation of any course in medicine is based on anatomy.

Physiology of the eye deals with the function of the eye, its capacities and limitations. The actual perception of light takes place in a well-delineated area called the *field of vision.* What is not seen beyond these boundaries is cataloged and stored in our visual memory center, so that we are not uncomfortable or handicapped by this imposition. Most eyes cannot form a sharp image on the retina without an internal adjustment made by focusing or by some external appliance such as lenses placed before them. There is a limit to how much detail the eye can resolve, its magnifying abilities being only ×15, considerably less than most microscopes. The spectrum of light that is sensitive to our retinal receptors is confined to specific wavelengths of light; the world of ultraviolet and infrared is invisible to ordinary perception.

Despite these limitations, the human eye is an extremely versatile instrument capable of seeing both in daylight and in dim light, registering colors, appreciating depth, and exercising rapid focusing adjustments. This chapter deals with the mechanisms that enable the eye to carry out these tasks.

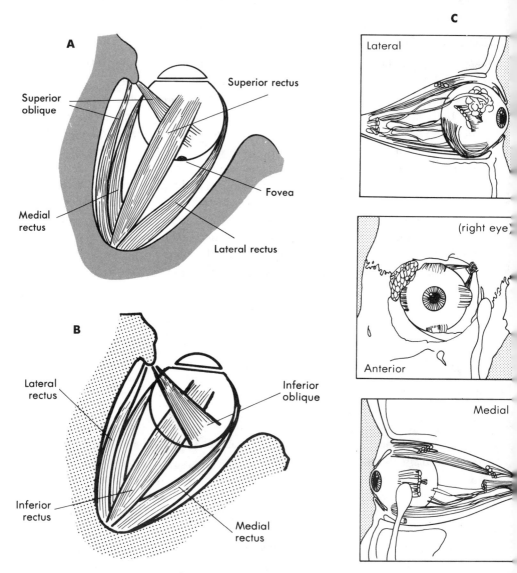

Fig. 1-19   A, Ocular muscles of the right eye viewed from above. Only the oblique muscles are inserted behind the center of rotation of the eye. All the recti muscles are inserted in front of the center of rotation of the eye near the limbus, where they are easily accessible for muscle surgery. **B,** Ocular muscles of the right eye viewed from below. **C,** The right eye viewed laterally, anteriorly, and medially.

ALIGNMENT OF THE EYES

In human beings, the two eyes work as though they were one, both projecting to the same point in space and fusing their images so that a single mental impression is obtained by this collaboration. Without this delicate balance, we would "see double," because two images would be formed by the independent action of each eye. In other words, *stereopsis* would be lost, since this faculty is totally dependent on the eyes' seeing in unison. The ability of the eyes to fuse two images into a single one is called *binocular vision.*

Binocular vision is dependent on an exquisite balance of motor and sensory function. The eyes must be parallel when looking straight ahead, and they must be able to maintain this alignment when gazing in other positions. Each impulse directing an eye to move in one direction must be equally received by the other eye. Further, the contraction of an eye muscle pulling the eye in one direction must be accompanied by an equivalent amount of relaxation of its opponent muscle. Without perfectly harmonious eye movement, binocular vision would be impossible, since eyes that do not move together do not see together.

Each eye must have good vision because a clear image and a fuzzy image cannot be fused. The fuzzy image is usually ignored by the brain (suppression). Each macula must have its projection straight ahead, so that the line of vision from each eye intersects at one point in space. Also, the field of vision from each eye must overlap (Fig. 1-20). Although we can see more with two eyes than with one, this difference is not great (about 35 degrees), because the majority of the field of vision from one eye overlaps the field from the other eye. Overlapping visual fields act as a locking device, forging our peripheral vision in place and thereby ensuring central fusion.

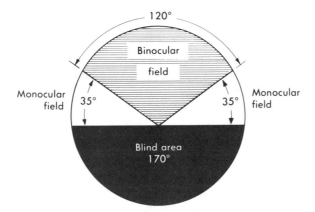

Fig. 1-20   Field of vision. Binocular field of vision (120 degrees) represents the overlapping field of vision from each eye.

FIXATION, OR LOOKING STRAIGHT AHEAD

Fixation involves the simple task of looking straight ahead toward an object in space. Fixation requires stability of the eyes and good monocular function. If the eyes are constantly moving, such as occurs with congenital nystagmus, the eyes can make only scanning motions about an object and never adequately see it in detail. Needless to say, if the ability to fixate becomes compromised by constant eye movements, then the visual acuity of the affected eyes is reduced. If the macula is damaged, fixation is difficult, because anything viewed directly ahead becomes enshrouded in relative darkness.

Fixation can be embarrassed without organic changes in the macula. Children with strabismus are often found to have poor vision in the turned eye. If a child has crossed eyes, we would think that double vision would occur, because the two eyes would not be directed to the same point in space (Fig. 1-21). However, children have a wonderful

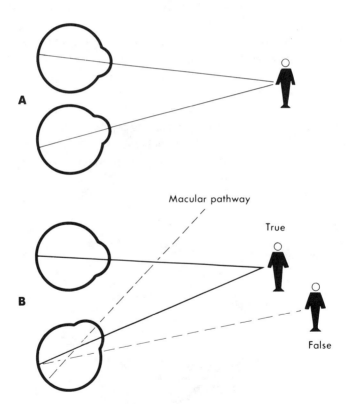

Fig. 1-21 **A,** Binocular vision (both eyes the same figure). **B,** One eye is turned in, resulting in double vision. In this case the figure is received by the macula of one eye and a point nasal to the macular of the turned eye. The projection of this nasal point results in the individual seeing two images instead of one of the same figure. This is an example of uncrossed diplopia, as seen in eso deviations.

faculty of completely ignoring the image in the turned eye to avoid confusion. It is this constant habit of actively suppressing the image in the turned eye that eventually leads to loss of vision, or *amblyopia.* In some of these children, in whom the suppression mechanism has become profound and the resultant vision very poor, foveal function becomes so depressed that a new point just outside the fovea is used. Such an eye can no longer see straight ahead, and the fixation pattern is described as *eccentric.*

FUSION, OR LOCKING IMAGES

Fusion is the power exerted by both eyes to keep the position of the eyes aligned so that both foveae project to the same point in space. Because fusion is a binocular act, it is easily disrupted by covering one eye. The eye under cover drifts to its fusion-free position. The amount of movement that the eye makes is a measure of the latent muscular imbalance kept in check by fusion, or the amount of heterophoria. *Heterophoria,* then, may be defined as the position the eyes assume when fusion is disrupted. The eye under cover may drift in, called *esophoria,* or may drift out, called *exophoria.* The eye may also drift up and down; this is called *hyperphoria* and hypophoria, respectively. Fusion may also be disrupted by placing a Maddox rod before one eye. The Maddox rod changes the size and shape of the image presented to the eye under cover so that fusion becomes impossible.

The power of fusion is measurable by prisms. For example, a 4-diopter prism is placed with the base toward the nose of an observer looking at a small letter placed 16 inches from the eye. The prism will displace the image before that eye in a direction toward its apex, and the eye moves outward to follow it because of the power exerted by the fusional reflex (Fig. 1-22, A). Now the prism is removed, and the uncovered eye

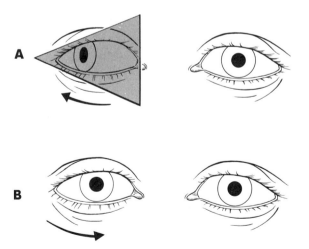

Fig. 1-22   A, The prism displaces the image toward its apex, and the eye moves outward because of the fusional reflex. **B,** When the prism is removed, the eye returns to its original position because of the fusional reflex.

returns to its original position again in response to the fusional reflex (Fig. 1-22, B). Normally, 20 to 40 prism diopters can be exercised by fusional convergence. The amount of fusion exercised with respect to divergence is less, being only 10 to 20 prism diopters. This is measured by using base-out prisms. Vertical imbalances are very difficult to overcome, as our eyes can overcome only about 2 to 4 prism diopters.

EYE MOVEMENTS

The primary position of the eyes is the straight-ahead position as they look at a point just below the horizon with the head held erect. Movement of the eye from the primary position to a secondary position occurs when the eyes are moved either horizontally or vertically. If the eyes are directed in an oblique position (up and in or down and in), they are said to be in a tertiary position.

The movement of one eye from one position to another in one direction is called a *duction*. In duction the fellow eye is either covered or patched. The movement of two eyes in the same direction is called a *version* (dextro, levo, sursum, and deorsum) (Fig. 1-23).

Eyes right: dextroversion
Eyes left: levoversion
Eyes up: sursumversion
Eyes down: deorsumversion

An outline of the functions of the extraocular muscles is given in Table 1-1. The medial and lateral rectus muscles have only one action—to move the eye horizontally. The other four muscles of the eye have auxiliary functions. When these secondary roles

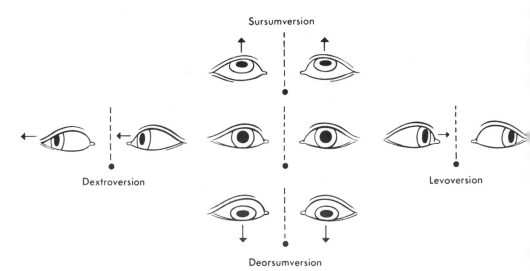

Fig. I-23 Version movements of the eyes. These are movements formed by both eyes working together.

Table 1-1   Actions of extraocular muscles

	Primary action	Secondary action
Medial rectus	Turns eye inward toward nose, or adducts eye	None
Lateral rectus	Turns eye outward toward temples, or abducts eye	None
Superior rectus	Elevates eye	Intortion Adduction
Inferior rectus	Depresses eye	Extortion Adduction
Superior oblique	Intorts eye	Depression Abduction
Inferior oblique	Extorts eye	Elevation Abduction

are used—assisting the lateral or medial recti to abduct or adduct—they are called *synergists* (Fig. 1-24).

The main function of the oblique muscles is to rotate the globe either inward *(intorsion)* or outward *(extorsion)*. Intorsion occurs when the eye rotates on its long axis so that the 12 o'clock position on the cornea moves toward the nose. For example, if a point on the cornea of the right eye moves inward from 12 to 1 o'clock, then intorsion

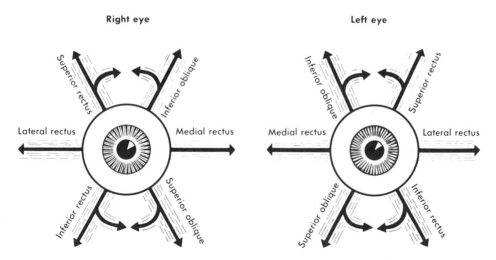

Fig. 1-24 Action of the extraocular muscles. The arrows reveal that the superior and inferior recti muscles function best as an elevator and a depressor, respectively, when the eye is abducted. The inferior and superior oblique muscles function best as an elevator and depressor, respectively, when the eye is adducted.

is said to occur because of the primary action of the right superior oblique muscle or secondary action of the right superior rectus muscle. Similarly, if the point on the right cornea moves outward from 12 to 11 o'clock, then extorsion is said to occur because of the primary action of the right inferior oblique muscle or secondary action of the right inferior rectus muscle.

Control centers for eye movements

The eyes move in response to our own volition, or they can move in a passive manner, such as in following a slow-moving target. Volitional eye movements are usually rapid, starting at high speeds and ending just as abruptly. Such movements occur with reading when words or phrases are quickly scanned, with an abrupt halt coming at the end of a section or a line. These voluntary eye movements are controlled from centers in the frontal lobe of the brain.

Whereas voluntary eye movements tend to be short and choppy, following or pursuit eye movements are rather slow, smooth, and gliding. The velocity of a following movement is entirely dependent on the speed of the object the eye is tracking. If the fovea is fixed on a moving target with an angular velocity (less than 30 degrees per second), the eye follows the target almost exactly. With greater speeds, following movement becomes difficult, and the smooth, gliding movement is replaced with an irregular, jerky movement. Pursuit movements are controlled from centers in the occipital lobe of the brain.

LOOKING TOWARD A CLOSE OBJECT

Vergence is the term applied to simultaneous ocular movements in which the eyes are directed to an object in the midline in front of the face. The term is usually applied to

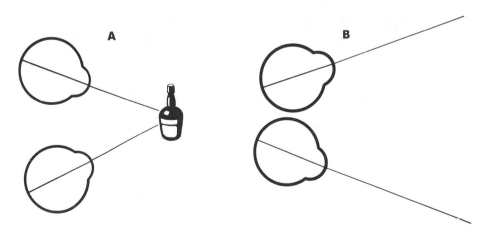

Fig. 1-25 A, Convergence. The eye is turned in toward the midline plane. **B,** Divergence. The eye is turned out away from the midline plane.

convergence, in which the eyes rotate inward toward each other, or to *divergence*, in which they rotate outward simultaneously (Fig. 1-25).

Convergence is invariably accompanied by narrowing, or constriction, of the pupils and by accommodation. The triad of convergence, pupillary constriction, and accommodation is often called the *accommodative reflex*, although in the true sense these movements are merely associated reactions (a synkinesis) rather than a true reflex. Each component of the triad facilitates fixation at near. The constriction of the pupil is the attempt by the eye to form a pinhole camera device so that a clearer image is seen; accommodation enables the object to be focused on the retina; convergence brings the eye inward toward the object of regard.

SEEING IN DEPTH

The ability to see in depth enables us to travel comfortably in space. Without it, we could not judge distances, estimate the size of objects beyond us, or avoid bumping into things. Without depth perception even the simplest of tasks would be difficult. We would be unable to reach accurately for our morning coffee, and passing a car on the highway would be more difficult. Fortunately, everyone has some depth perception, whether they possess one eye or two. A one-eyed person learns to estimate depth with monocular clues (Figs. 1-26 and 1-27). He knows that the speck in the distance that becomes a huge train standing beside him in the station has not grown larger but has merely come closer. Other clues besides the size of the object also assist. The train tracks spread from a point and become parallel, the color of the train changes from a misty blue-gray to dark green, the sound increases, and when the train is alongside, one can feel the heat. There are many monocular clues that facilitate depth perception. They include the following:

- Magnification. Well-recognized objects, if they become larger, are deemed to be nearer
- Confluence of parallel lines to a point—for example, railway tracks
- Interposition of shadows
- Blue-gray mistiness of objects at a great distance
- Parallax. If two objects situated at different points in space are aligned and the head of the observer is moved in one direction, the nearer object will appear to move in the opposite direction

However, a monocular person, if removed from familiar surroundings, would have great difficulty in judging distances because of a lack of any intrinsic depth-perception mechanism. For example, a one-eyed pilot would create a hazard because of the difficulty he or she would experience in maneuvering in space without the normal monocular clues.

Stereopsis is a higher quality of binocular vision. Each eye views an object at a slightly different angle, so that fusion of images occurs by combining slightly dissimilar images. It is the combination of these angular views that yields stereopsis. The same method is used in photography in making three-dimensional pictures. The stereoscopic picture is taken at slightly different angles and later viewed that way.

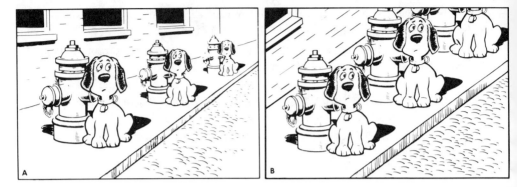

Fig. 1-26 A, Artist has drawn the picture with proper depth perspective. Monocular clues include decrease in size of dogs and confluence of lines toward a point. **B,** Artist has ignored the usual monocular clues so that our appreciation of depth and size is erroneous. The second dog appears larger than the first, although both are the same size.

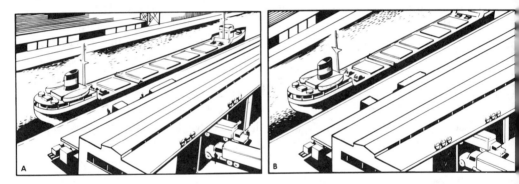

Fig. 1-27 A, The scene is drawn using normal monocular clues of distance, thereby giving it perspective. **B,** The same scene is drawn without regard to the normal impressions of distance. Therefore, the scene loses its perspective.

ACCOMMODATION, OR FOCUSING AT NEAR

Any object moved from a distance to about 20 feet in front of an observer can still be seen clearly without accommodation. This distance is called the *range of focus.* However, if the object is brought closer than 20 feet, the eye must continuously readjust to keep the image of the object clearly focused on the retina. This readjustment requires an increase in the power of the eye and is brought about by an automatic change in the shape of the lens in response to a blurred image (Fig. 1-28). This zoom-lens mechanism in the eye is very active in children, since they are able to see a small letter in clear focus only 7 cm from the eye, whereas an adult of 55 years can focus no closer than 55 cm. The *range of accommodation* is the distance in which an object can be carried to-

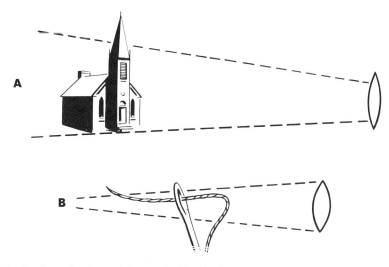

Fig. 1-28 A, Crystalline lens of the eye is thin for distant objects. **B,** Crystalline lens accommodates for near objects by becoming thicker. This increases its effective power.

ward an eye and be kept in focus. The power of accommodation of an eye is the dioptric equivalent of this distance. By age 75 years this power is zero.

Both the range and the power of accommodation are measured quite easily. When the full spectacle correction is worn, it is merely the closest point at which an accommodative target (such as a small letter) can be seen clearly. It is usually equal in both eyes. The range of accommodation is measured in centimeters, whereas the power is converted to diopters (Table 1-2).

Table 1-2   Accommodation and near point of the normal eye

Age	Near point in centimeters	Available accommodation in diopters
10	7	14
20	9	11
30	12	8
40	22	4.5
45	28	3.5
50	40	2.5
55	55	1.75
60	100	1
65	133	0.75
70	400	0.25
75	Infinity	0

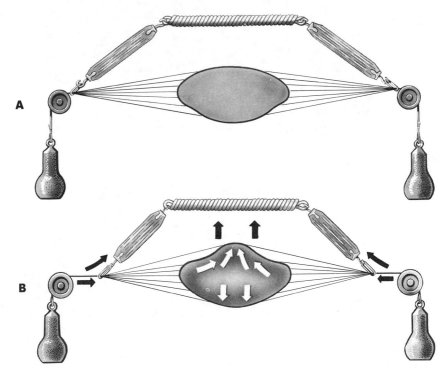

Fig. 1-29 Adjustment of the crystalline lens by accommodation. When the zonular ligaments are relaxed, the inherent elasticity of the lens causes it to increase in thickness and therefore increase in power. (Redrawn from Krug WFS: Functional neuro-anatomy, New York, 1953, The Blakiston Co.)

This stimulus for accommodation is a blurred image on the retina. As an object is moved closer to the eye, the rays of light entering the pupil must be continuously converged. This change in focusing power of the eyes is brought about by active contraction of the ciliary muscle. The contraction of this muscle causes the zonular fibers of the lens to relax, which in turn allows the lens of the eye to change its shape (Fig. 1-29). In the child and the young adult, the lens can be molded, and it increases its power by becoming thicker and increasing the curvature of its anterior space. In an adult the ability of the ciliary muscle to effectively contract declines with age, and the lens becomes harder and less malleable with advancing years.

The decline in accommodation with age, presbyopia, is remedied with reading glasses or bifocals. It usually becomes apparent by the age of 45 years.

TRANSPARENT PATHWAY FOR LIGHT

For light to effectively stimulate retinal receptors, clear media for transmission are necessary. One of the prime functions of the eye is maintenance of the transparent pathway for light (Fig. 1-30).

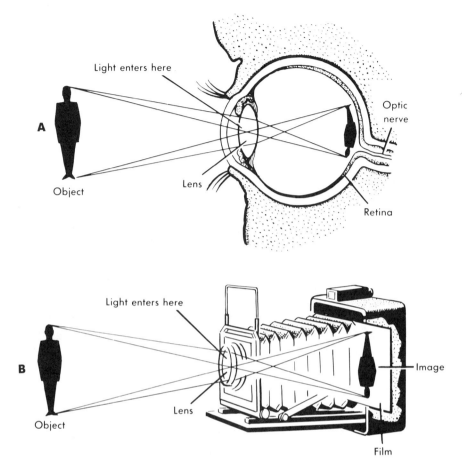

Fig. I-30 The eye is like a camera. Light must have a clear pathway to be clearly focused on the sensory receptors of the retina or the film of a camera.

The cornea is the window through which light rays pass on their way to the retina. Its cells and collagen fibers are so arranged that light can pass through it with a minimum of diffraction and internal reflection. The cornea is transparent because its fibrils are arranged in a parallel manner and are tightly packed and separated by less than a wavelength of light. When the cornea is swollen, this arrangement is distorted, and the cornea becomes hazy. The cornea contains no opaque substances, such as blood vessels, that would mar its clarity. It receives its nourishment from perilimbal vessels, the tear film, and the aqueous humor. The cornea is kept shiny and lubricated by tears that keep its surface moist and fill out any irregularities in its superficial epithelium.

The most important factor in maintaining corneal transparency is the ability of the cornea to keep itself relatively dehydrated. If a section of cornea is placed in isotonic saline solution, it becomes hydrated, opaque, and edematous. On the other hand, if the sclera is dehydrated, it becomes transparent.

The cornea has an active, pumplike mechanism located in the corneal epithelium and endothelium that enables it to keep itself relatively dehydrated. Damage to the corneal epithelium or endothelium results in the cornea's becoming hydrated and swollen. Swelling of the cornea, whether localized or diffuse, always results in a loss of transparency. If the swelling (that is, corneal edema) is located centrally, then vision will be blurred. In acute angle-closure glaucoma, the sudden rise in intraocular pressure causes epithelial edema. The individual droplets in the epithelium break up white light to its colored spectral components, and the patient complains of seeing colored halos around lights. The rainbow we see after a storm is similarly explained; it is merely the effect of suspended water droplets in air breaking up white light.

Transparency is also aided by the ability of the corneal epithelium to rapidly regenerate. The corneal epithelium, by sliding over defects and regenerating its cells, can cover a large abrasion within 24 hours, and without leaving a scar. If Bowman's layer or the corneal stroma is damaged, repair takes much longer, and a permanent scar forms.

The aqueous humor is in constant circulation, flowing from the posterior chamber through the pupil to the anterior chamber, where it leaves the inner eye proper through the trabecular meshwork, the canal of Schlemm, and the aqueous veins (Fig. 1-31). If the exit of aqueous humor from the eye is blocked, the volume of fluid within the eye

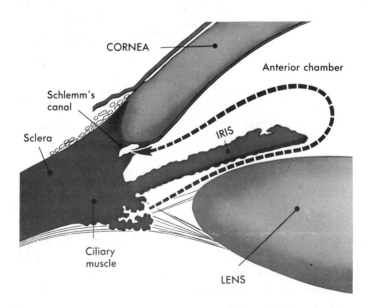

Fig. 1-31 Flow of aqueous humor. Aqueous humor is largely produced by the ciliary processes in the posterior chamber and flows into the anterior chamber and leaves the eye through the canal of Schlemm.

increases; and because the coats of the eye are relatively nondistensible, the pressure within the eye also increases.

As light travels through the eye, the next structure it encounters is the iris, with its central round opening, the pupil. The iris is the shutter mechanism of the eye, controlling the amount of light entering the eye in the interest of clear vision. If the amount of available light is excessive, the pupil constricts by the action of the sphincter muscle of the iris to reduce excessive light or glare. If the illumination is poor, then the pupil dilates to increase the amount of light entering the eye. Other factors also control the size of the pupil. Emotional arousal (for example, fear, anxiety, or erotic stimulation) tends to dilate the pupils. Pain in the body dilates the pupil. The pupils are generally large in young, blue-eyed, and myopic persons, and they tend to be smaller in brown-eyed and older persons. The pupils normally are round in shape and equal in size. If a light is directed to one eye, both pupils constrict. The constriction of the pupil on the side toward which light is directed is called the *direct light reflex*, whereas the pupillary response in the fellow eye is called the *consensual light reflex*.

As light passes through the pupil, the next structure it encounters is the lens. The lens of the eye is a biconvex structure, completely surrounded by a capsule. It has only a single layer of epithelial cells under its anterior capsule, which does not significantly interfere with its transparency. Like the cornea, it contains no opaque tissue such as blood vessels, nerve fibers, or connective tissue. It is nourished solely by the aqueous humor that bathes it.

Lens material in a child is very soft and puttylike in consistency. However, with age the lens becomes harder, especially centrally. As new lens fibers form, they envelope the previously existing fibers, compressing them and pushing them into a compact unit toward the center. Thus growth of the lens is not accompanied by an increase in size after puberty but by a compression and tight lamination of the older fibers. The central hard portion, called the nucleus, usually becomes well formed by the age of 30 years.

There are two main parts of the lens: the dense center, or nucleus, and the surrounding cortex. This arrangement offers an optical advantage in making the total refractive power of the lens greater than if the index of refraction were uniform throughout.

The *vitreous body* is located directly behind the lens and occupies two thirds of the entire volume of the eye. It is a transparent gel, that is, a viscous fluid midway in composition between a solid and a liquid. Functionally and metabolically the vitreous is relatively inactive. If the lens and cornea are compared with the lenses of a camera, the vitreous body is the space before the film. Frequently with age, the gel breaks down in part, becoming liquid. This degeneration of the vitreous gives rise to the often-heard complaint of seeing spots before the eyes.

Once light has left the vitreous, the last great transparent structure of the eye, it finally strikes the retina, which contains all the receptors sensitive to light.

The *retinal receptors* are divided into two different populations of cells—the rods

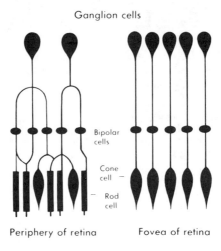

Fig. 1-32 Rods and cones of the retina.

and the cones (Fig. 1-32). The rods are far more numerous (approximately 125 million) than the cones (approximately 6 million) and function best in dim illumination (scotopic vision). Without rods, night blindness occurs. Individuals affected with a disorder involving a selective loss of rod cells can see very well during the day as long as the illumination is high, but under conditions of poor illumination, as in movie theaters or darkrooms, they are totally unable to adapt and behave as though blind. The cones function best in daylight (photopic vision) and mediate straight-ahead vision and color vision. A selective loss of cone cells results in a loss of visual acuity and an inability to perceive colors. This duplicity of function among the retinal receptors is easily demonstrated by entering a darkroom illuminated only by a red light. The rods are relatively insensitive to red and therefore do not lose their function with this type of lighting. At first everything appears quite dark, then hazy, and finally the definite shapes of objects at the sides come into view as the rods begin to function. The total duration for dark adaptation to be completed is about 30 minutes. Darkrooms (for example, photography darkrooms and x-ray rooms) are usually equipped with a red light because it allows the cones to function and straight-ahead vision to be preserved while enabling the rods to become dark adapted.

The process of dark adaptation requires a neural change in the rod cells that is rapid, and a chemical change in the outer segments of the rod cells that is slow (at least 30 minutes). The chemical change is a complex process requiring the synthesis of the rod pigment called *rhodopsin.* Rhodopsin, or visual purple, forms under conditions of dark adaptation and is destroyed by light. Therefore, it is continuously being used and restored. One of the main components of rhodopsin is vitamin A, found in carrots and other vegetables. Vitamin A deficiency causes night blindness, but the corollary that an excess of vitamin A will help the eyes is not true. The cones also contain a pigment called *iodopsin.*

Because the fovea contains no rods, but only a concentration of specialized cones, it is found that when the eye is fully dark adapted, there is a central loss of vision. Although visual acuity is not as good in this state, the perception of light is enhanced because the rods have a lower threshold for light sensitivity than the cones. Visual information in the form of light strikes the photoreceptors and this sets off a chain of events that leads to the process of seeing. Impulses from the photoreceptors are carried to the bipolar cells and then in turn to the ganglion cells. The site of connections between cells is called the *synaptic zone.* The information from the ganglion cells then travels via axons through the optic nerves, the chiasm, and the optic tract to synapse with cells in the lateral geniculate body. Impulses are then carried by axons to the occipital cortex for the processing of the information.

RETINAL IMAGES

Retinal images, once formed, persist for a very short period of time. They are called *positive afterimages.* Normally one is not aware of this persistence of retinal images because the eyes take up a new gaze that obliterates the former afterimage. In making movies, sensation of motion, or flow, is produced only when the film speed of the camera is sufficiently fast to enable fusion of the images produced by the moving frames on the film. If the camera is slowed, flickering occurs because there is a time gap between the afterimage of the first sequence and that of the next.

Negative afterimages also occur. This is commonly witnessed as a dark spot appearing before the eyes after one has been photographed with the use of a flashbulb. The high-intensity light exhausts the retinal receptors, and they become unresponsive to further light stimulation for seconds after. Negative afterimages are employed in a test for strabismus to determine the direction of fixation. High-intensity flashes placed in a vertical or horizontal position will produce a dark line of the same dimension as a flash. This line can be drawn by the patient. If fixation is central and straight ahead, the reproduction is exact. If the fixation pattern is eccentric, then the picture drawn will be decentered by an amount equal to the degree of eccentric fixation.

INTRAOCULAR PRESSURE

The normal intraocular pressure is between 13 and 19 mm Hg. These numbers are derived by measurements using a tonometer and indicate the pressure in the eye that will not normally cause damage to the intraocular contents. Individual eyes respond to intraocular pressures differently. Some can tolerate pressures in the high 20s, and some will have damage to the optic nerve with lower pressures.

Transient and physiologic variations occur in the intraocular pressure. With respiration, these variations in intraocular pressure can amount to 4 mm Hg, whereas changes of 1 to 2 mm Hg occur with each pulsation of the central retinal artery. The changes with pulse beat are nicely demonstrated on tonographic recordings, which always show a sawtooth type of graph in rhythm with the beats of the pulse. Throughout the day the intraocular pressure can vary as much as 3 to 4 mm Hg, the maximum pressure being found around 6 AM. In a glaucomatous eye the fluctuations in diurnal pressures can be 6 to 8 mm Hg per day or even greater.

The pressure in the eye is largely dependent on the amount of aqueous humor secreted into the eye (1 to 2 cu mm per minute) and the ease by which it leaves. The flow of aqueous into the eye varies with the general hydration of the body. In dehydrated states, the amount of aqueous produced will decrease, and so will the pressure within the eye. On the other hand, if large quantities of fluid are quickly ingested, the amount of aqueous secreted will increase. Forced hydration is used in the water-drinking test, since a rise of 8 mm Hg or more 45 minutes after drinking 1 liter of water is suggestive of glaucoma. The drug acetazolamide (Diamox), used in the treatment of glaucoma, acts by reducing the volume of aqueous produced.

The rate of fluid exit from the eye, or its facility of outflow, is the most important single factor regulating the intraocular pressure. Glaucoma is rarely caused by an increase in aqueous production but is invariably linked to a decrease in the facility of outflow.

There are three primary methods of occluding the outflow channels of the eye. In open-angle glaucoma (the most common type) the diameter of the openings of the trabecular meshwork becomes narrowed, thereby increasing the resistance of fluid flow (Fig. 1-33). This situation is analogous to a drainage system in which the final common drain tube is suddenly reduced to a tube of only half its diameter at the very end. The amount of water leaving the system should be very small, and the pressure in the tube in front of the narrowing would be very high.

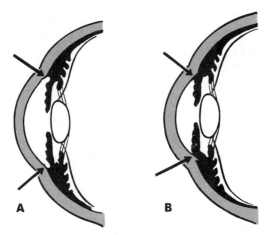

Fig. 1-33 Glaucoma. **A,** Open-angle glaucoma. The obstruction to aqueous flow lies in the trabecular meshwork. **B,** Closed-angle glaucoma. The trabecular meshwork is covered by the root of the iris.

In secondary glaucoma the trabecular meshwork becomes blocked. The obstructing matter can be in the meshwork and may consist of red blood cells with hyphemas, tumor cells, pigment, and debris. In addition, the obstructing matter may cover the meshwork itself in the form of scar tissue, or anterior synechiae between the iris and the angle structures. These adhesions, which are commonly formed following a severe iritis, an episode of angle-closure glaucoma, or a central retinal vein occlusion, produce a severe and intractable glaucomatous state.

Another method of occluding the outflow channels occurs with pupillary block, as typified in primary angle-closure glaucoma. In eyes predisposed to this condition, the angle formed by the root of the iris and the angle structures is quite narrow. If the pupil in such an eye is dilated, the iris tissue, which folds up like an accordion on dilation, abuts against the angle structures and partially blocks it. In addition, the aqueous humor in the posterior chamber has difficulty circulating through the anterior chamber. Therefore the pressure in the posterior chamber increases and bows the iris to a more forward position, obstructing even further the already compromised exit channels of the eye. This process occurs quite suddenly, and the eye does not have the chance to accommodate itself to the high intraocular pressures reached. As a result the eye becomes red, the cornea edematous, the pupil fixed and dilated, and the patient complains of considerable pain. Angle-closure glaucoma constitutes an ocular emergency and is relieved by a peripheral iridectomy, where a small portion of the peripheral iris is removed to facilitate transfer of fluid between chambers. This procedure can be performed in the operating room; it is more commonly performed in the office with the use of either the Argon or Yag lasers.

TEARS

The surface of the eye is kept moist by tears formed by the lacrimal gland and the accessory lacrimal glands located in the superior and inferior fornices. Evaporation is minimized by a thin film of oil secreted by the meibomian glands over the layer of tears. Tears function to keep the globes moist and to fill in the interstices between the corneal epithelial cells to provide a smooth, regular corneal refractive surface.

Only 0.5 to 1 ml of tears is produced during the day; minimal tears are produced at night. About 50% of the tears are lost through evaporation, and the rest are carried to the superior and inferior puncta on the medial aspect of the upper and lower lids and are drained through the nasal lacrimal duct into the inferior meatus of the nose (Fig. 1-34).

The tear film is composed of three layers (Fig. 1-35). The outermost layer consists of a lipid or fatty layer, mostly cholesterol esters, and is extremely thin. This layer is secreted by the meibomian glands. It acts to prevent evaporation of the underlying aqueous layer. The central layer is chiefly aqueous, with some dissolved salts as well as glucose, urea, proteins, and lysozyme. This layer is secreted by the lacrimal glands. The third layer is a very thin mucous layer lying over the surface of conjunctiva and cornea. This layer is secreted by specific cells of the conjunctiva called *goblet cells*. This mucous

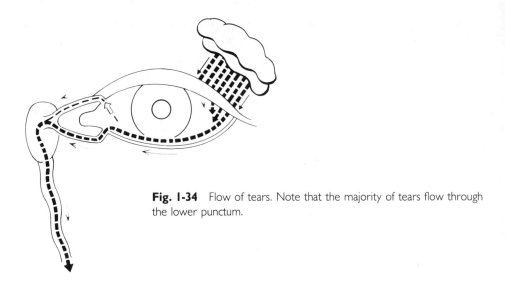

Fig. I-34 Flow of tears. Note that the majority of tears flow through the lower punctum.

layer is important in the stability of the tear film. Tear film abnormalities may arise in association with a number of clinical problems in the aged and particular problems related to contact lenses.

Tear formation occurs as a result of psychic stimuli and reflex stimuli. Reflex stimuli involve uncomfortable retinal stimulation by bright lights or irritation of the cornea, conjunctiva, and nasal mucosa. The amount of tear production is measured by the Schirmer test. This test is performed by simply placing a strip of filter paper 5 mm wide into the lower fornix for 5 minutes; over 10 mm of wetting indicates normal function.

COLOR VISION

The cones of the human eye are thought to contain three different photosensitive pigments in their outer segments. These pigments act by absorbing light of certain definite wavelengths according to their period of vibration. The pigments of the cones are sensitive to red, green, and blue, the three primary colors of light. (This is not to be confused with the three primary colors of red, blue, and yellow, as found in the paint mixing field and used by artists.) Other colors are formed by mixtures of these pigments.

Color depends on *hue, saturation,* and *brightness.* An object will have a particular hue because it reflects or transmits light of a certain wavelength. The addition of black to a given hue produces the various *shades.* Saturation is an index of the purity of a hue. The brightness of an object depends on the light intensity. Today we can experiment with all these aspects of color by turning various knobs of a color television set to achieve the variations of hue, saturation, and brightness.

Color vision defects are believed to arise from a deficiency or absence of one or more visual pigments. Clinically, persons with abnormal color vision fall into three major categories. The *trichromat* possesses all three cone pigments and has normal color

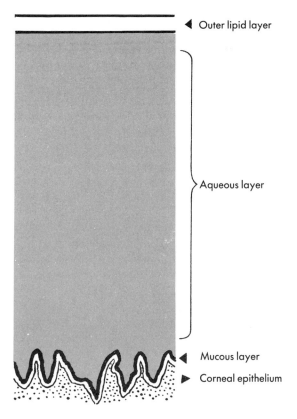

◀ Outer lipid layer

Aqueous layer

◀ Mucous layer
▶ Corneal epithelium

Fig. I-35   Three-layer structure of the tear film.

vision. Those of us who have been tested and found normal belong to this category. The *anomalous trichromat* has a partial deficiency of one of the three cone pigments. He or she may have (1) *protanomaly*—deficiency in sensitivity to the first color (red), and poor red-green and blue-green discrimination; (2) *deuteranomaly*—deficiency of one pigment mediating green, and poor green-purple and red-purple discrimination; or (3) *tritanomaly*—deficiency of the cone pigment for blue, and blue-green and yellow-green insensitivity. The *dichromat* has a complete deficiency in one cone pigment but preserves the remaining two cone pigments. The person may have (1) protanopia, in which red is absent, (2) deuteranopia, in which green is absent, or (3) tritanopia, in which blue is absent. The *monochromat* has only one cone pigment.

The degree of color deficiency is determined by a series of plates or charts. The most common test used is the Ishihara color plate test, in which the ability to trace patterns on a multicolored chart is measured.

The milder deficiencies (anomalous trichromatism) are by far the most common, with red and green deficiency predominating. This type of color deficiency has a sex-linked recessive mode of inheritance and affects approximately 8% to 10% of all males and less than 1% of females.

2　Ophthalmic history-taking

There are two types of patients entering an ophthalmologist's office: the patient who desires a routine ocular examination combined with a refraction and the patient with symptoms of an ocular disorder. Unfortunately, it is often impossible to distinguish between the two on the basis of a history. Each patient, then, must be questioned as though one expects to find some ocular disease.

ORGANIZATION OF A HISTORY

The history should be subdivided to maintain organization. Many charts have the organization stenciled or printed on them. Regardless of the charting method used, an ophthalmic history should include the following:

Chief complaint
History of present illness
History of past health
    Significant medical illnesses
    Previous eye disorders
    Previous surgery, both ophthalmic and general
Medications employed presently and their duration of use
Allergies
    Inhalants
    Contactants
    Ingestants
    Medications
Family history of ocular disorders
    Myopia
    Strabismus
    Glaucoma
    Blindness
Occupation
    Type of work
    Industrial hazards

Although many complaints are strictly ocular in nature, others are a manifestation of poor general health or emotional problems. Occasionally a patient may be taking medication that he or she feels has no effect on the eye and will not reveal this aspect of his history unless specifically asked. For example, a patient with a duodenal ulcer may be given propantheline bromide (ProBanthine), an atropinelike drug that inactivates the ciliary muscle. Such a patient would consult an ophthalmologist because of difficulty seeing at near or a feeling of dryness of the eye.

CHIEF COMPLAINT

The chief complaint constitutes the headlines of any ophthalmic history. In a sentence or two one should write down the main reason for which the patient has come for advice and help. In this context the prime question should be direct, simple, and forthright. *How do your eyes trouble you?* The patient may reply concisely or give a long, rambling account of various symptoms. If the patient cannot focus thoughts on the main issue after repeated questioning, one should record what he or she regards as the most serious problem among the patient's symptoms. Commonly described chief complaints are *pain, loss of vision, eye fatigue,* and *blurred vision for near.* One must then proceed to pin down the specifics of the complaint such as date of onset, cause, and duration.

HISTORY OF PRESENT ILLNESS

After the chief complaint is recorded, the patient should be questioned about the main symptoms with greater detail. When did the problem begin and under what conditions? In other words, what was the patient doing when something was first noted to be amiss? Was the onset slow or rapid in development, and did it affect one or both eyes? Once the onset of the patient's symptoms has been recorded, their development and progress should be noted. What did the patient do after it began? Did he consult a doctor, a friend, or a pharmacist? Did he take any medications internally or place any in the eye? Did the symptoms appear to become worse or to abate? Was the problem relieved by taking any medication or stopping a particular activity? In other words, what aggravated it and what made it better? The patient should be asked how long he has had a particular symptom and whether it tends to recur.

To aid the dissection of a symptom, the pertinent points regarding the most common ophthalmic complaints are reviewed next.

Loss of vision

Very few patients will actually state that they have lost vision, unless, of course, they have become blind because of some unfortunate tragedy. Most patients complain of blurred vision and state this problem in terms of a limitation of function. Blurred vision may assume many forms.

Blurred vision secondary to an error of refraction. Hazy, foggy, or blurred vision, if it occurs at a particular distance, usually indicates a refraction error. The myope cannot see in the distance, and the hyperope may have difficulty at near. It is the patient with astigmatism who has difficulty seeing both in the distance and at close range. However, even with astigmatism, poor visual acuity is not evenly distributed, since this type of patient will generally see better at close range because of the magnification afforded by proximity. Most patients with refractive errors have a specific visual disability limited to specific activities.

Blurred vision for close work. A patient whose vision is blurred for close work is usually a presbyope over 40 years of age and may complain of an inability to read the stockmarket report or a number in the phone book.

Blurred vision for distance work. In this instance the patient is not apt to be a young adult for whom a fresh diagnosis of myopia is about to be made. If the patient is in school, most often he will complain of inability to see the blackboard. If the patient drives an automobile, he will state that road signs appear to be quite fuzzy, especially at dusk. Occasionally a patient will recognize this problem by noting that the television set appears fuzzy only to him. With regard to television, mothers often become very alarmed when their children sit close to a television screen. This is not usually a symptom of myopia because children enjoy sitting close to the screen for two reasons. First, they enjoy the magnification because big things are easier to view, and, second, the closer they are to the screen, the greater is their sense of involvement with the story being told.

Blurred vision secondary to organic disease. The patient with organic disease has difficulty seeing things at all times regardless of the activity. If the patient has a cataract or macular degeneration, he will be limited in both the distance (driving) and at near (reading). The patient with a cataract sees as though looking through a frosted glass window, and the patient with macular disease finds things missing when he looks straight ahead, so that he must look at them askew.

Loss of central vision. With loss of central vision the patient discovers that he is unable to see clearly straight ahead but that he has retained his peripheral vision (Fig. 2-1). When looking at a face he may state that the face appears gray or indistinct, whereas the background around the face appears to be clearer. Such a patient commonly sees better in dim illumination. The visual acuity in the affected eye is usually quite poor. This symptom, if sudden in onset, usually means a disorder of the macula or the optic nerve.

Distorted vision. Distortion of vision is most commonly a sign of macular edema. The patient with this symptom usually complains that objects appear minified and slightly fuzzy and that their contours are curved rather than straight. Visual distortions are also common in patients, such as high myopes, who wear very thick lenses.

Night blindness. The patient with night blindness finds difficulty in seeing things in the early evening, and his difficulty becomes much worse as night falls. Such a patient behaves as though blind in movie theaters, darkrooms, and so forth, yet he can see quite clearly straight ahead in daylight. Eventually the patient suffers visual field restrictions, which makes driving and later ordinary ambulation quite difficult even during the

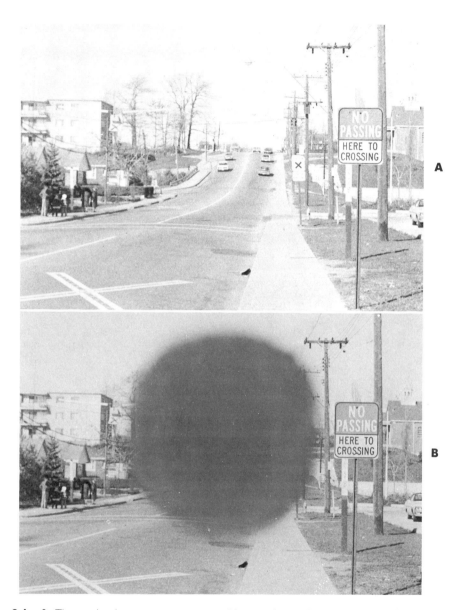

Fig. 2-1 **A,** The road as it appears to a person with normal central and peripheral fields of vision. **B,** Loss of central field. The central field of vision is indistinct, whereas the peripheral field of vision remains clear.

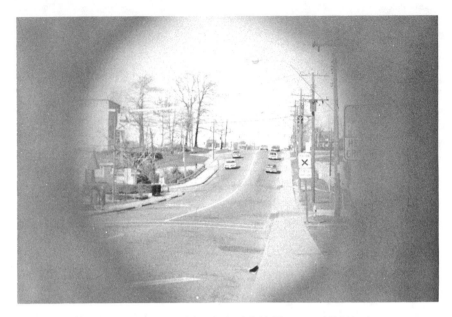

Fig. 2-2 Restricted peripheral visual field. The central field is clear.

day (Fig. 2-2). This symptom may be a manifestation of retinitis pigmentosa or vitamin A deficiency.

Transient gray-outs or blur-outs of vision lasting several seconds in one or both eyes. Although this symptom appears to be inconsequential, it often is of great importance. These obscurations of vision may be a symptom of papilledema (swelling of the disc as a result of increased intracranial pressure), carotid insufficiency, and arteriosclerosis.

Inability to see to the right or to the left. This symptom follows a profound field loss in which the patient loses half his field of vision. Such a patient, when reading the visual acuity chart, sees letters on half the chart only and sees them clearly to the 20/20 line of the unaffected side. Usually the patient has difficulty in any visual tasks, such as driving, reading, or even ordinary ambulation (Fig. 2-3). When this occurs on the same side in both eyes, one has to be suspicious of brain involvement of the opposite side.

Ascending veil. The patient may see a dark shadow ascending like a fog arising in his lower field of vision. This symptom is frequently an ominous indicator of a retinal detachment from above (Fig. 2-4).

Headaches

Headaches are a headache for all medical personnel. Commonly the patient with a headache has been referred by the family doctor, who, unable to find an organic cause for the complaint, has referred the patient to an ophthalmologist for further assessment. Unfortunately, most headaches are not caused by a refractive error or a disorder within

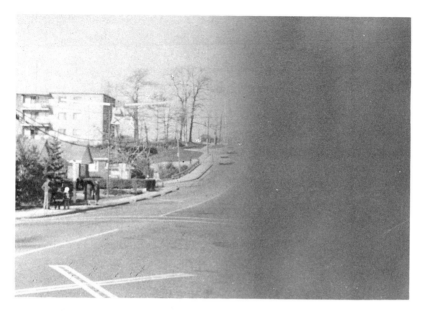

Fig. 2-3 Restriction of vision in the right visual field.

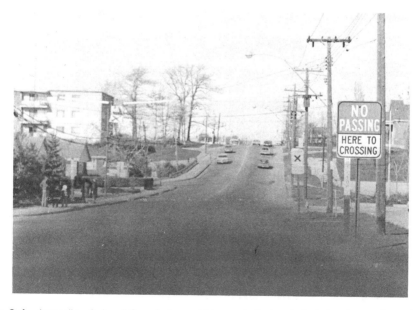

Fig. 2-4 Ascending dark veil from below, which may indicate a retinal detachment from above.

the eye, and the ophthalmologist must lamely report to the family doctor that there appears to be no ocular cause for the patient's headaches. Although the symptom of headache is difficult to evaluate, it must be treated with respect, since this complaint may be indicative of many sinister conditions, such as severe hypertension or brain tumor. Of importance in the assessment of any headaches are the following:

1 *Family history of headaches.* In many of the vascular headaches, such as migraine, a positive family history is frequently obtained.

2 *Onset and duration.*

3 *Severity.*

4 *Associated symptoms.* In this regard the ophthalmic assistant is really searching for other findings associated with the headache. For example, the patient with a migraine headache sees an aura before the onset of the headache. This aura usually consists of flashing of lines in zig-zag formation, extending from the central area to the periphery and lasting approximately 20 minutes. Other important associated symptoms that should be noted are nausea, vomiting, blackouts of vision, fainting spells, weakness of an arm or leg, numbness of the fingertips, and difficulties with coordination.

5 *Relationship of the headache to visual activity.* Do the headaches follow prolonged periods of close work, or do they appear when the patient rises in the morning? Obviously, headaches caused by errors of refraction will not appear at night, during sleep, or on awaking.

6 *Character of the headache and its location.* A notation should be made of the nature of the patient's headache, whether it is vicelike, throbbing, or dull, and also of its location, that is, in or above the eyes, or in the temple regions.

Asthenopia

Asthenopia is a wastebasket term denoting a number of sensations accompanying uncorrected refractive errors and problems in ocular motility. Included in this ocular wastebasket of symptoms are the complaints of (1) general eyestrain, (2) eye fatigue after reading, (3) pulling sensations, (4) inability to focus, (5) heaviness of the lids after reading, (6) sensitivity to sunlight or fluorescent light, (7) tendency to fall asleep after reading one or two pages, and (8) burning, itching, and watering of the eyes with reading.

Besides refractive errors, these symptoms may be a result of chronic conjunctivitis, allergy, lack of tears, an emotional disorder, or fatigue. The patient with asthenopic complaints is apt to be vague and elusive in describing his symptoms. Because the disability tends to be minor, lapses of memory are frequent, and the patient is often reduced to repeating that "my eyes just don't feel right" (Table 2-1).

Red eye

The most common cause of a red eye is acute conjunctivitis. The salient features of conjunctivitis are discharge, pain, and blurred vision.

Discharge. The discharge of conjunctivitis can vary from being profuse and watery

Table 2-1   Asthenopic symptoms

SYMPTOMS INDICATING URGENCY	POSSIBLE CAUSES
Pain in the eye	Chemical burn
	Flash burn to cornea
	Keratitis
	Glaucoma
	Iritis
	Temporal arteritis
	Retrobulbar neuritis
Sudden loss of vision	Macular degeneration
	Cortical retinal artery occlusion
	Retinal detachment
	Central retinal vein occlusion
	Retrobulbar neuritis
Transient loss of vision	Carotid artery disease
	Migraine
	Papilledema
	Severe hypertension
Diplopia	Myasthenia gravis
	Thyroid disorders
	Diabetes
	Third nerve palsy from any cause
Ptosis	Third nerve palsy
	Diabetes
	Myasthenia gravis
Flashes of light	Retinal detachment
Trauma	Blow out fracture of the orbit
	Hyphema

SYMPTOMS REQUIRING PROMPT ATTENTION	POSSIBLE CAUSES
Discharge and matting of the lids in the morning	Conjunctivitis
Red eye	Any external disease of the eye
Swelling of the lids	Bilateral blepharoconjunctivitis
	Acute allergies
	Thyroid disease
Halos around lights	Angle closure glaucoma
	Cataracts
Blurred vision in the elderly	Macular degeneration
	Cataracts
	Ischemic optic neuropathy
Persistent tearing in one eye	Dacryocystitis
	Blocked tear duct
	Entropion, extropion
	Trichiasis
	Chalazion
	Bell's palsy
Enlarging nodule on the lid	Basal cell carcinoma
Foreign body sensation	Corneal foreign body
	Corneal abrasion
	Herpes simplex keratitis

Continued

Table 2-1   Asthenopic symptoms—cont'd

SIGNIFICANT SYMPTOMS THAT SHOULD BE SEEN AS SOON AS POSSIBLE	POSSIBLE CAUSES
Gritty feeling	Dry eye syndrome from any cause whatsoever
	Conjunctivitis
	Ocular irritation—dust, wind, ultraviolet lights
Headaches	Often tension
	Hypertension
	Brain tumor
	Migraine, cluster headaches, etc.
Blurred vision for distance in an adult	Diabetes
	Cataract
	Macular edema
Spots before the eye	Retinal tear
	Vitreous detachment
Pain behind the eye	Sinus disease
	Thyroid disorders
	Orbital tumor (rare)
	Aneurysm of the carotid artery (rare)
Eruption on the skin	Atopic allergy
	Seborrhea
	Herpes zoster
	Drug reaction

to being rather scant or purulent. During the day, of course, the discharge tends to drain and is wiped away with handkerchiefs and other tissues, but during the night it tends to accumulate and dry. Thus the patient with conjunctivitis complains that his lids are stuck together in the morning, the lashes being matted together in the dry discharge.

Pain. Normally there is no pain with simple conjunctivitis unless the cornea is involved. A secondary keratitis is a common accompaniment of conjunctivitis, especially if the offending organism is *Staphylococcus aureus.* The patient usually complains of a sandy or scratchy feeling or of having the sensation of a foreign body in his eyes.

Blurred vision

Because the clarity of the optical media is not affected by conjunctivitis, visual loss is not a prominent complaint in this condition. However, because of the discharge over the surface of the cornea, the vision in the affected eye may be hazy. Occasionally such a patient even complains of seeing halos about lights.

In cases of conjunctivitis it is very helpful to gain information regarding the source of the infection. Inquiry should be made into the presence of a similar disorder appearing in relatives or friends. Detection of the source of the infection may be very important, especially in crowded institutions such as orphanages or army barracks, where in-

Table 2-2   Differential diagnosis of common causes of the inflamed eye

	Acute conjunctivitis	**Acute iritis**	**Acute glaucoma**	**Corneal trauma or infection**
Incidence	Extremely common	Common	Uncommon	Common
Discharge	Moderate to copious	None	None	Watery and/or purulent
Vision	Normal	Slightly blurred	Marked blurring	Usually blurred
Conjunctival injection	Diffuse	Mainly circumcorneal	Diffuse	Diffuse
Pain	None	Moderate	Severe	May be pain or irritation
Cornea	Clear	Usually clear	Steamy	May be corneal abrasion, foreign body, or ulcer due to virus or bacterium
Pupil size	Normal	Small	Large	Normal
Pupillary light response	Normal	Poor	Poor	Normal
Intraocular pressure	Normal	Normal	Elevated	Normal
Smear	Causative organism	No organisms	No organisms	No organisms unless taken directly from cornea in case of bacterial ulcer

From Vaughn D, Cook R and Asbury T: General ophthalmology, Los Altos, Calif, 1965, Lange Medical Publications.

fection can travel through an entire group. It is also important to ask the patient if treatment has been started by either the family physician or the patient himself.

Other causes. The red eye is also a manifestation of *acute iritis* and *acute narrow-angle glaucoma*, although the incidence of these two conditions is far less than that of acute conjunctivitis. The diagnosis of acute glaucoma can virtually be made over the telephone. The onset of this condition is quite sudden and dramatic, with the entire triad of pain, loss of vision, and congestion of the globe occurring within a matter of 30 minutes. The pain of acute glaucoma, unlike that of conjunctivitis, is quite intense, and the patient may have associated nausea and vomiting. Also, the visual loss is profound, and frequently the vision is reduced to hand movements or counting fingers. The only real distinguishing feature between acute glaucoma and acute iritis, in terms of symptoms, is the difference in the onset of the two conditions. Iritis takes hours or days rather than minutes before it becomes fully developed.

The differential diagnosis of the common causes of an inflamed eye is outlined in Table 2-2.

Diplopia, or double vision

The patient with true diplopia states that he sees two objects instead of one. This symptom occurs when there is an acquired loss of alignment of the eyes, so that each eye does not project to the same place in space. Loss of ocular alignment is a common finding in children with strabismus. However, children with strabismus do not see double, because they are capable of suppressing the vision in one eye to avoid the confu-

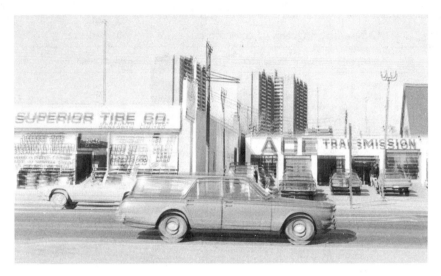

Fig. 2-5 Double vision. The images are just slightly displaced vertically.

sion of double images. Adults are not as adaptable as children and quite disabled by double vision (Fig. 2-5). They have faulty spatial orientation and projection and complain of dizziness, inability to walk straight, and inability to reach accurately toward an object in space. If the diplopia results from the loss of alignment of the eyes, then covering one eye will always eliminate the second image.

Occasionally the patient may have monocular diplopia. With monocular diplopia

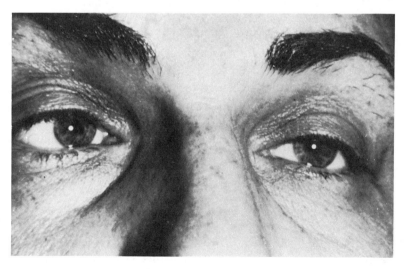

Fig. 2-6 Recent onset of paralysis of right lateral rectus muscle. Right eye has turned in.

the double vision persists when one eye is closed. It is important to make this distinction in the history. Binocular double vision is always caused by the development of a weak or paralyzed extraocular muscle. The loss of alignment results from the fact that an opponent muscle carries the eye over to one side, being unopposed by the palsied muscle. For example, if the right lateral rectus muscle becomes paralyzed, the right medial rectus muscle would carry the eye inward toward the nose (esotropia) (Fig. 2-6).

Monocular diplopia is quite uncommon and may be caused by an extra pupil or cataracts, or it may appear in the recovery phase after strabismus repair.

Floating spots and light flashes

Virtually everyone has seen, at some time or another, small spots before the eyes. They may appear singly or in clusters; they may be punctate or linear; they may travel with the movements of the eye or against them. These floaters are most apparent when the illumination is high and when one is gazing at a clear surface. The most common situations in which they are seen include looking up at a clear summer sky, gazing against a blank white wall, and reading.

These floaters are usually caused by the formation of small particles in the vitreous body and generally are innocuous. However, floaters may, on occasion, be indicative of a more serious derangement within the eye. They may be caused by cells in the vitreous from an active iridocyclitis, or they may be secondary to a retinal tear, to hemorrhage, or to a detachment.

Tearing

Tearing as an isolated event occurs most commonly as a result of a blockage of the nasolacrimal duct. In infants it results from failure of the duct to become completely canalized. Although tearing is most often a sign of a blocked nasolacrimal duct, it can also be caused by congenital glaucoma, foreign bodies in the cornea, or inturned lashes. Every child with tearing should be assessed carefully.

In adults tearing is a less specific symptom. It may occur as a result of entropion, chronic conjunctivitis, allergy, or obstruction of the nasolacrimal duct. In taking a history of a patient whose primary complaint is tearing, one must note (1) the duration of tearing, (2) whether it appears to come from one eye or both, and (3) associated findings, such as redness of the eye or discharge.

PAST HEALTH, MEDICATIONS, AND ALLERGIES

The patient should be asked about his general health at present and its status in the past. In particular, diabetes, hypertension, cardiac disorders, and arthritis should be mentioned. Many systemic disorders have ocular manifestations. If a positive history is obtained, the ophthalmologist can direct the examination with greater purpose.

Equally important is obtaining a history of any medications the patient may be taking. Often the patient will not know the name of the medication but will refer, for example, to a green tablet and a yellow tablet, as though the color of the pill or tablet were its identifying mark. When possible the ophthalmic assistant should call the patient's pharmacy to identify the exact name of the medication the patient is taking. If this is not feasible, the patient should be asked the purpose of the medication. Usually most patients are aware of their general function and will state that the pill is for reducing swelling in the legs or relieving high blood pressure.

One should also inquire into the presence or absence of allergies. In general, five types of allergic responses should be inquired about:

1. Allergy to drugs (taken internally or applied topically)
2. Allery to inhalants (dust, pollens, and so forth)
3. Allergy to contactants (cosmetics, woolens, and so forth)
4. Allergy to ingestants (food allergies)
5. Allergy to injectants (tetanus antiserum)

FAMILY HISTORY

It is helpful if inquiry is made into the familial history of the more common ocular defects. In particular, the presence or absence of such familial diseases as myopia, strabismus, and glaucoma should be asked about. A negative family history does not rule out a genetic familial propensity. Many patients really do not know the ocular status of their relatives, whereas others, being very family proud, are reluctant to confess to any weaknesses in the lineage.

Common familial disorders

Migraine
Retinitis pigmentosa
Retinoblastoma
Color blindness
Nystagmus
Albanism
Sickle cell anemia
Choroideremia
Keratoconus
Von Recklinghausen's disease (Elephant man's disease; neurofibromatosis)
Marfan's syndrome
Diabetes
Hereditary macular degeneration (Stangardt's disease)

TIPS IN HISTORY TAKING

A systematic order in taking an adequate history should be followed:

1. Identify the chief reason the patient has presented for an eye examination.
2. Identify any secondary reasons or problems the patient has that are referable to the eye.
3. Identify any systemic or general illness the patient presently has and any medication being taken.
4. List past ocular disorders or operations.
5. Determine if the patient is wearing contacts or spectacles, and if so, how old they are and when the last eye examination occurred.

6. Be succinct but also go into detail with any specific ocular problem that arises. General questions, such as time and duration, family involvement, and so on, regarding any abnormality may be important.
7. Record any previous therapy and the response.

SUMMARY

The analysis of the importance of symptoms is a difficult task, because a symptom is merely an expression of disordered function. It depends not only on the patient's condition but also on his ability to define his trouble with lucidity. Exaggerations, distortions of complaints, irrelevancies, vagaries, and lapses of memory tend to lead the examiner astray. A good historian should not interpret for the patient. If a given history is not precise, a vague statement of the patient's actual complaints should be recorded. The interpretation of the history, combined with the physical findings, is the responsibility of the doctor, who arrives at a final diagnosis.

3 Skills to learn for an ophthalmic examination

ASSESSING VISUAL ACUITY

Standards have been established for visual acuity charting. It has been found that the normal eye can distinguish two points separated by an angle of 1 minute to the eye. By convention, most visual acuity charts are constructed so that the sections of a letter subtend 1 minute of arc. Each letter is printed on squares made up of five parts in each direction so that the whole letter that is to be identified subtends a 5-minute angle to the eye (Fig. 3-1).

Visual acuity (VA) should be assessed both with and without glasses, using a standard eye chart. Each eye should be tested independently. In testing visual acuity, one should always use an opaque card or an occluder. If the examiner uses his or her own hand or the patient's hand, there may be small gaps between the fingers through which the patient may sometimes look and thus a false reading will result. To obtain the best corrected vision, one should have the patient wear his distant glasses or bifocals if he has them.

Visual acuity is determined by the smallest object or line that can be clearly seen and distinguished at distance. The commonly used Snellen charts consist of letters carefully designed to subtend this 5-minute angle of the eye at specified distances (Fig. 3-2). Generally speaking, 20 feet or 6 meters has been considered a practical distance for assessing vision, and the charts have been calibrated with this in mind. At 20 feet the distant rays of light from an object are practically parallel, and very little effort of accommodation is required. In rooms that are shorter than 20 feet, mirrors may be used to achieve the required 20-foot distance. In some cases, charts are proportionately reduced in size to compensate for a room with a shorter working distance.

Results of vision testing are expressed as a fraction. The numerator denotes the distance the patient is from the chart letter, and the denominator denotes the distance from the chart at which a person with normal vision can see the chart letters. For example, if a person reads the 20/20 at 20 feet, then his visual acuity is recorded as 20/20 (VA = 20/20). If he reads a 20/60 line at 20 feet his visual acuity is recorded as 20/60

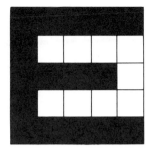

Fig. 3-1 The letter E. Each section of the letter subtends 1 minute of arc. The whole letter subtends 5 minutes of arc.

(VA = 20/60). This means that the individual can see at 20 feet a letter that a person with normal vision can see at 60 feet.

In the Western hemisphere, visual acuity charts are generally designated in feet, whereas in Europe the metric system is employed. In order of best to worst vision, visual acuities are recorded as 20/15, 20/20, 20/25, 20/40, 20/50, 20/60, 20/70, 20/80, 20,200 and 20/400. To test visual acuity, one should place the chart on a light or uncluttered wall that has no windows nearby. The chart should be fastened at eye level. The recommended illumination on the wall chart is 10 to 30 candles, but many offices use projected types of vision charts or retroilluminated charts. Illumination in the room should not be less than one fifth the amount of illumination on the chart. In assessing vision, an occluder is gently placed over one of the patient's eyes without exerting any pressure. A line read is recorded as 20/20, or whatever the case may be. If one or two letters are missed on the line, this may be recorded. For example, if the patient sees a 20/20 line but misses one letter, visual acuity should be recorded as 20/20 minus 1.

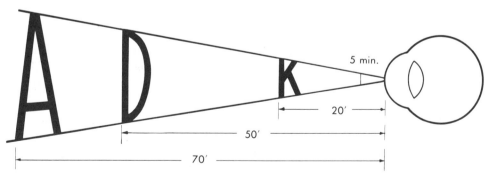

Fig. 3-2 Each letter on the visual acuity chart subtends a 5-minute angle to the eye independent of the distance.

Table 3-1   Conversion table of visual acuity

Meters	Feet
6/6	20/20
6/7	20/25
6/9	20/30
6/12	20/40
6/18	20/60
6/24	20/80
6/30	20/100
6/60	20/200
6/90	20/300
6/120	20/400

If the vision is poor, then the largest letter (usually 20/400, large E) then the following are the systems of recording the vision. The patient is taken closer to the wall chart until the large E is identified. For example, 4/200 indicates that the patient was 4 feet from the 20/200 letter. If he cannot identify the letter as close as 1 foot, the examiner then holds his or her fingers before that patient's eye in good light and the vision is recorded at the farthest distance at which the fingers can be counted. For example, if the patient can accurately count the number of fingers the examiner is holding at 3 feet away, this is recorded as "counting fingers at 3 feet." If the patient cannot distinguish fingers as close as 1 foot, the examiner should wave a hand in front of the eye. If movements of the hand are perceived by the patient, the vision is recorded as "HM," or hand movements. If the patient cannot even detect hand movements, the room is darkened, a test light is shone in the eye from the four quadrants, and the patient is asked to point in the direction of the light. If the patient can accurately point to the light, vision is recorded as "light projection." If he cannot distinguish the position but is able to just detect the light, visual acuity is recorded as "light perception." If the patient is unable to detect light at all, vision is recorded as "absent light perception" or blind.

Illiterate persons and preschool children may be tested by charts made up of numbers or pictures or by Landolts broken rings. In the commonly used E test, the child points to the direction of the E either with his finger or with a hand held cut out E. With the Landolts broken ring test the child merely identifies where the break in the ring occurs. There may be flashcards with identifiable pictures for the illiterate and the child that can be held in the hand and correspond with the picture on the chart.

For near vision, the examiner holds the near vision card at normal reading distance (about 14 inches) and the individual reads the smallest print that he can identify. It may be recorded as 14/14. Some near charts are designated in Jaeger numbers. Jaeger was an ophthalmologist who recorded the smallest print as J1 and ranged size to larger

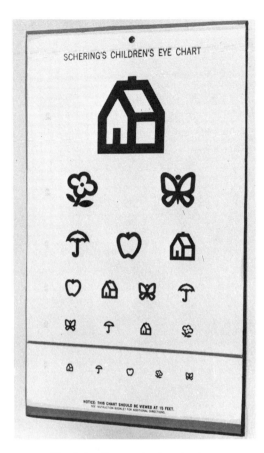

Fig. 3-3   Picture visual acuity chart.

numbers. Alternatively, some reading cards are made up with point numbers after printers' points, where N.5 is the normal print size that an average person can see at 14 inches.

When visual acuity is tested, the following points should be noted.

1. A false idea of visual acuity will be obtained if an isolated letter is presented to the patient rather than a line of letters. This is particularly true in individuals with amblyopia, who may have 20/40 or 20/50 vision when tested with isolated letters and only 20/200 when asked to identify letters in a series.

2. Each eye must be tested independently, because some patients are unaware of an amblyopic eye or an eye with defective vision.

3. There can be a difference with recognition of letters in the same line. The letter L is considered the easiest letter in the alphabet to identify and B the most difficult. The letters T, C, F, and E are progressively more difficult.

4. Vision should always be tested with and without the patient's glasses so that the comparison between the two can be made. The best vision is usually with glasses.
5. In children, visual acuity testing should not be prolonged and fatiguing.
6. If the child cannot comprehend the organization of the E game, he should receive practice at home. Parents can be given a small E printed on a card or an E cube to teach the child to play the game of visual acuity testing.
7. In all visual acuity measurements, one should note when there is any consistent pattern in the letters missed by the patient. For example, failure to see the nasal half of the chart may be indicative of a serious field defect, with loss of vision of half the visual field of each eye.
8. If both eyes are tested together, it is usually found that each eye reinforces the other so that binocular vision tends to be slightly better than the vision of each eye tested separately.
9. The observer should watch the patient so that he is not partially closing his eye or "squinting." This causes a decreased pupillary aperture and thus allows only the central rays to enter the eye, giving the individual better vision than the patient would normally have. The eyes must be kept wide open.
10. The observer should watch the patient to be certain that he is not peeking around the occluder.

Use of the pinhole disk

When the pinhole disk is placed before the eye, it eliminates peripheral rays of light and improves contrast and generally improves vision to almost within normal limits. This is important if the patient has a refractive error that is eliminated by the pinhole. The pinhole disk thus serves to differentiate visual loss caused by refractive errors from poor vision resulting from disorders of the eye or brain. In the latter conditions, vision is not improved when a pinhole disk is placed before the eye.

Dynamic visual acuity

Visual acuity measured in an office setting is quite artificial. The eyes are steady, the body is still, and the target is immobile. In real life, as we walk down the street, the body is in motion. The body is displaced both forward and vertically, and the object of regard is rarely still. We look at things in action. This type of acuity is sometimes called *kinetic vision* or *dynamic visual acuity.*

Kinetic vision or moving vision cannot be measured, but it is known that acceleration reduces acuity. The faster one travels, the more the vision degrades. Body displacement spoils good vision, for example, trying to read on a truck with poor shock absorbers. Fast eye movements are also detrimental to seeing clearly. It is impossible to see a tennis serve travelling over 100 miles an hour. Therefore the coach's pronouncement of "keep your eye on the ball" is a misnomer in fast tennis or other such sports.

Contrast sensitivity

Another aspect of vision is contrast gradient visual acuity. This is a measure of the acuity when hampered by poor contrast. A person can have 20/20 Snellen acuity and complain of poor vision. Snellen acuity measures only an individual's ability to see small high-contrast images. A visual contrast test can assess the entire spectrum of images in contrast. An individual with cataracts or night blindness may see well in daytime but see poorly at night or on cloudy days, when there is low contrast.

Glare testing

Visual acuity may degrade considerably in the presence of bright light. This is particularly true if there are opacities in the media, such as with a posterior polar cataract. A number of glare test devices are available on the market (TVA, BAT, Eye Con) that create a dazzle effect that identify the individual whose vision is reduced by glare. The brightness acuity test (BAT test) delivers three controlled degrees of light when the eye is visualizing a Snellen target. Vision with opacity of the ocular media, cornea, lens, posterior capsule, and vitreous, when under the effect of bright light, will degrade considerably and produce a true visual acuity measurement in ambient lighting.

Macular photostress test

The macular photostress test is used to detect macular dysfunction such as cystoid macular edema, central serous retinopathy, and senile macular degeneration. Under bright light conditions, patients with these disorders are slow to recover acuity. Normal recovery to bright light is 0 to 30 seconds, but it can be prolonged to over 1 minute when macular disorders are present.

COLOR VISION ASSESSMENT

Defects in color vision may be congenital or acquired. Congenital color defects occur in about 8% to 10% of males and only in 0.4% of females. This defect is transmitted through the female and appears predominantly in the male. Acquired color blindness may occur after diseases of the optic nerve or central retina.

Congenital color blindness may be partial or complete. In the completely color-blind patient the visual acuity is reduced and the patient usually has nystagmus. All colors appear gray, but of different brightness. Fortunately, this form of color blindness is rare. The partial form is a hereditary disorder transmitted through the female, who usually is unaffected. In the majority of patients the color deficiency is in the red-green area of the spectrum. With the deficiency in red, this color appears less bright than for the normal individual and thus mixtures of colors containing red are often confused with other colors. Deficient color vision of the red-green variety may pose problems for drivers, sailors, pilots, textile designers, and others for whom distinguishing colors is an important function. Absence of blue color is very uncommon.

Tests for color blindness are multiple and varied and consist of matching colored balls or yarns, the red-green lantern test, and the most popular test, isochromatic plates.

In clinical practice it is sufficient to test with pseudoisochromatic plates, such as the Ishihari plates. More scientific approaches to color vision testing are available but are not generally used for routine clinical practice.

Ishihara test plates

The Ishihara book consists of a series of pseudoisochromatic plates that determine color blindness and particularly red-green blindness (Fig. 3-4). These plates are viewed by the observer under good illumination. They consist of dotted numbers of one color against the background of another. If color vision is normal, the dots, arranged as a numeral, stand out and the patient can read the appropriate number. A person with normal sight may see one number, whereas a color-blind person viewing the same plate would interpret the dots as forming a completely different number. For patients unable to read numbers, plates are present in the album with colored winding lines that may be traced by finger.

Hardy-Rand-Ritter plates

This series of plates includes plates for yellow-blue color blindness as well as red-green color blindness. The background is a neutral gray on which a series of circles, crosses, and triangles of color are superimposed. These designs are present in higher and lower saturations of color to detect the degree of color vision deficiency. With this color vision test, not only can a graded diagnosis be made (mild, medium or severe), but also the yellow-blue defects may be differentiated as well as the red and green.

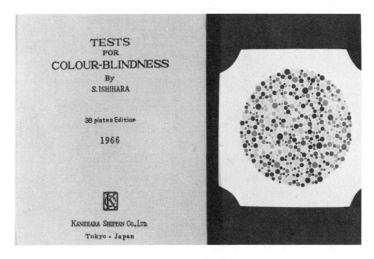

Fig. 3-4 Ishihara's test for color blindness.

DEPTH PERCEPTION

Depth perception is the highest quality of binocular vision, because it provides the individual with judgment concerning depth, based on the coordinate use of two eyes together. A prerequisite for depth perception is good vision in each eye, overlapping visual fields, and normal alignment of the eyes in all positions of gaze. Four main tests that are available are the fly test, the Wirt stereo test, the Worth four-dot test, and the biopter test.

Fly test

The patient is provided with Polaroid lenses and asked to touch the wings of a fly. If the patient has depth perception, the wings will appear to stand out before the picture (Fig. 3-5). The patient will have a gross stereopsis of approximately 200 seconds of arc.

Wirt stereo test

Animals in three lines are shown to young school-aged children or even to preschoolers who seem able to grasp the idea of the test. If all three lines of animals are correctly selected, the patient has stereopsis of approximately 100 seconds of arc.

The raised rings in nine frames are shown to older children, adults, or even to younger children, if possible, depending on the alertness of the child. If all nine groups are correctly selected, it may be assumed that the patient's normal stereopsis is approximately 40 seconds of arc. In this portion of the test, two groups must be missed in

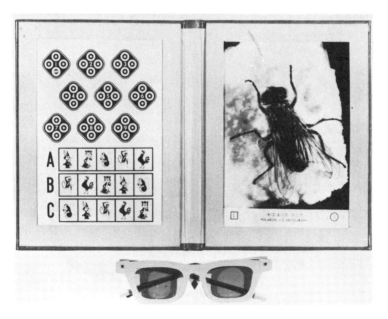

Fig. 3-5 Wirt and fly tests for depth perception.

succession for the examiner to stop the test. For example, if the patient correctly selects groups 1,2,3,5,6 and misses group 4, 7, and 8, number 6 would be counted as the patient's maximum amount of stereopsis.

Worth four-dot test

In the original Worth four-dot test one white disk, one red disk, and two green disks are presented to the patient who is wearing spectacles with a red-free green lens before one eye and a green-free red lens before the other eye. This allows both of the patient's eyes to see the white disk. However, the eye covered with the red lens will see in addition to the white disk only the red disk. The eye covered with the green lens will see in addition to the white disk only the two green disks. The patient is then asked to report the number of disks seen. If four disks are seen, both eyes are functioning together. If three disks are seen, then the eye behind the green lens is seeing the two green and one white, while the eye behind the red lens is suppressing. If two disks are seen, then the eye behind the red lens is seeing the red and white disk while the eye behind the green lens is suppressing. If five disks are seen, another problem is indicated—the eyes are not fusing together and muscular imbalance is suspected.

EXAMINATION OF THE EXTERNAL OCULAR STRUCTURES, LID, AND LACRIMAL APPARATUS

One should begin the external examination by systematically noting the symmetry of the orbits, lid margins, conjunctiva, lacrimal apparatus, sclera, cornea, iris, pupil, and lens. (Fig. 3-6). On grossly examining the eye itself, the examiner uses a penlight and holds up the upper eyelid. Points to be noticed are:

- Is the eye white or red?
- Are the pupils reacting normally?
- Is there a bright corneal reflex?

The patient should be instructed to look to the right, to the left, and up and down. Both eyes should be examined in this way.

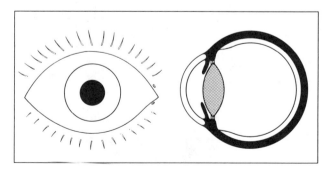

Fig. 3-6 Examination of the anterior segment includes an assessment of the lids, puncta, conjunctiva, sclera, cornea, anterior chamber, and lens.

Symmetry of orbit

In proptosis (exophthalmos), in which one eye protrudes, the upper lid is often re-tracted and there is exposed sclera above and below the cornea (Fig. 3-7). Another method of determining the presence of proptosis is to stand above the seated patient, draw his upper eyelids upward, and note which eye appears to bulge the most. One may also record the degree of proptosis with an instrument called an *exophthalmometer* (Fig. 3-8).

Eyelids

Cilia or eyelashes are hairs on the margins of the lids. They are located in two rows, totalling about 100 to 150 cilia on the upper lid and half that number on the lower lid. The bases of these cilia are surrounded by sebaceous glands (glands of Zeiss). Infections of these glands result in a common sty. The average life of the cilium is from 3 to 5 months, after which it falls out and a new one grows in to take its place. If the cilium is pulled out, the new one replacing it reaches full size in about 2 months. If the cilia are cut short, as is sometimes done preceding surgery on the eye, regrowth is rapid and lashes may appear normal in a few weeks.

Lid margins

The lid margin should be observed for any redness, scaling, or discharge indicative of blepharitis. The position of the lid margin should also be noted. It should be tight

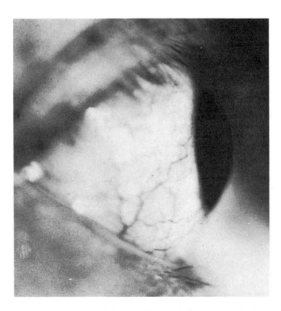

Fig. 3-7 Proptosis of the eye. Note the lid retraction and the exposed sclera above and below the cornea.

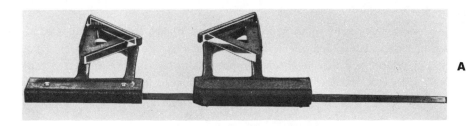

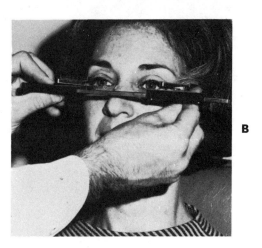

Fig. 3-8   A, Hertel exophthalmometer. **B,** Measurement of eye protrusion.

against the globe and not sag outward (ectropion) or fold inward (entropion). The punctum on the medial aspect of the lower eyelid should not be visible without depressing the lower eyelid. The more common conditions of the lid margin are stys, chalazions, and growths.

Conjunctiva

The bulbar conjunctiva is readily visible. The caruncle is seen as a fleshy mound of tissue at the inner canthus. The palpebral conjunctiva of the lower eyelid is seen by depressing the lid while the patient looks toward the ceiling. The palpebral conjunctiva lining the upper lid and tarsal plate can be visualized only by everting the upper lid.

Lacrimal apparatus

The tear film that covers the surface of the eye is composed of three layers:
1. A superficial oily layer derived from the meibomian glands and the sebaceous gland of Zeiss, which prevents evaporation of the underlying tear layer
2. The tear film, the middle layer, secreted by the lacrimal gland and the accessory glands of Frause and Wolfing

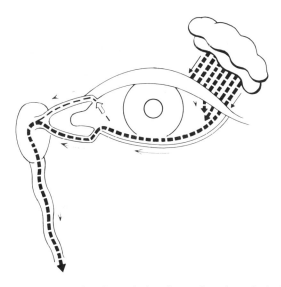

Fig. 3-9 Flow of tears. Note that the majority of tears flow through the lower punctum.

   3. The deepest layer, the mucoid layer, secreted by the goblet cells of the conjunctiva

Tears are normally carried from the lacrimal gland situated laterally to the nasal side along the lower lid margin. When they reach the opening of the lower lid, the punctum, they drain into the nasolacrimal duct and finally into the nose (Fig. 3-9). Blinking spreads the tear film over the eye but also moves the tears toward the punctum with each blink. Tears contain albumin, globulin fractions, and an antibacterial enzyme called *lysozyme*. Tear production may decrease 30% or more in a person over 50 years of age. The condition of dry eyes may be established.

   Distention and chronic inflammation of the lacrimal sac may cause a small, smooth elevation of the lacrimal fossa between the inner canthus and the nose. Pressure inward on this area will cause the contents of the lacrimal sac to be expressed by way of the punctum onto the conjunctiva. It should be noted whether the contents of the lacrimal sac are tears, mucus, or purulent material. This may be infected or may be a mucocele of the lacrimal sac.

   Deficiency of tears is best measured by the Schirmer test (Fig. 3-10). A standardized filter paper 3 mm by 20 mm is inserted in the unanesthetized lower fornix of each eye at the junction of the middle and nasal third of the lower eyelid margin. With the eyes gently closed, these strips become moistened by the tears. The amount of paper moistened can be measured with a millimeter ruler and recorded.

   Normally, the lacrimal gland, under the irritation of a piece of filter paper, produces sufficient tears to wet at least 10 mm of the paper in 5 minutes. Tear production of less than 10 mm indicates a dryness of the eye, and xerosis or keratoconjunctivitis

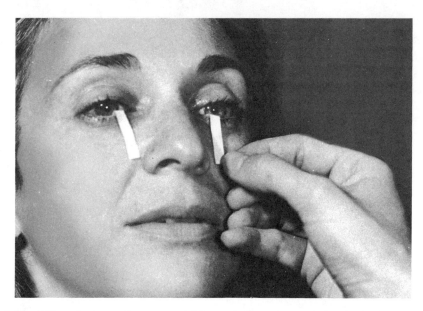

Fig. 3-10 Schirmer's test to detect tear deficiency. A filter paper strip is permitted to remain in contact with the eye for 5 minutes.

sicca may be present. Less than 3 mm of wetting is grossly pathological. Lack of tears may cause dry eyes, burning or sandy or gritty feeling. This test is important for contact lens wearers to determine whether there are sufficient tears for the comfortable wearing of contact lenses.

A variation of the Schirmer test is accomplished by placing an anesthetic drop into the conjunctival sac before the Schirmer paper is inserted. The purpose of the topical anesthetic is to eliminate the reflex tearing caused by the paper itself.

EVERSION OF THE UPPER EYELID FOR FOREIGN BODIES

The palpebral conjunctiva lining the upper eyelid can be visualized only by everting the upper lid. Foreign bodies are often located under the eyelid. In addition, the palpebral conjunctiva under the eyelid will often show papules and follicles indicating disorders such as viral and allergic conjunctivitis.

To evert the upper eyelid, one should grasp the lashes of the upper lid between the thumb and the index finger and turn the eyelid over a toothpick or applicator. The latter should be applied at the lid fold while the *patient looks downward.* By looking downward, the patient relaxes the levator muscle. Eversion of the upper eyelid is an important skill to learn in the management of foreign bodies and the identification of viral and allergic conjunctivitis.

EXAMINATION OF THE SCLERA AND CORNEA
Sclera

The normal sclera is visible beneath the conjunctiva as a white, opaque, fibrous structure. Blue discoloration of the sclera may be normal in a very young child because of the sclera's thinness and the underlying prominence of the dark choroid. In the elderly, the sclera may appear yellowish because of the presence of fat and other degenerative substances.

Cornea

The cornea is the first and most powerful lens of the optical system of the eye. The radius of curvature of the average cornea can be measured with a keratometer in a central region. The reaction of the cornea to disease is unique in that the cornea is vascular and cannot fend off infection easily. The surface layer of the cornea, the epithelium, is easily disrupted but fully regenerates when injured by flash burns, contact lens injuries, abrasions, and superficial corneal foreign bodies. Most infections and injuries involve only the corneal epithelium. The underlying Bowman membrane shows some resistance to pathologic conditions. It may be easily destroyed and produce scar tissue. Descemet's membrane is quite strong and highly resistant. The endothelial cells may die and never regenerate. The neighboring endothelial cells enlarge and fill in the gap of dead cells. Thus total endothelial cell count in any given area becomes important

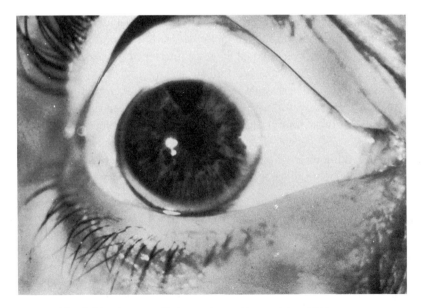

Fig. 3-11   Arcus senilis in a patient with a peripheral iridectomy.

and can be viewed by specular microscopy. If the cornea becomes swollen, it loses its shape and transparency and develops corneal clouding. This swelling can occur with acute glaucoma, with loss of function of the endothelial cells, producing bullous keratopathy.

In children, the corneal diameter should not exceed 11 mm. Corneal enlargement of 12 mm or greater is strongly indicative of congenital glaucoma. In the elderly, a white ring is frequently present near the corneal periphery. This creamy white ring is the result of the deposition of fat and is called arcus senilis (Fig. 3-11). The cornea is normally free of blood vessels. If blood vessels are present, they are a pathologic condition and indicate disease. Corneal edema can often be seen with the naked eye because of its characteristic ground-glass appearance. Corneal opacities may be detected by oblique illumination with a small flashlight.

Corneal sensation may be tested with a small wisp of cotton directly applied to the cornea. Comparison of the corneal reflexes of the two eyes is most useful. Loss of corneal sensitivity follows the herpes simplex virus and disorders that involve the fifth (trigeminal) nerve.

USE OF FLUORESCEIN AND ROSE BENGAL STAINS

Fluorescein is an ocular stain used to show defects and abrasions in the corneal epithelium. The pooling of fluorescein on small corneal defects is best seen by means of ultraviolet or cobalt blue light for illumination. This causes the fluorescein to fluoresce. There is a danger with fluorescein in solution form. It becomes easily contaminated with *Pseudomonas aeruginosa,* which appears to flourish in fluorescein. Sterile dry fluorostrips in which fluoroscein has been impregnated are available to prevent this complication. The fluorescein strip should be moistened with a drop of saline and applied to the lower fornix. This will cause liquid fluorescein to replace the tear film. The ulcer or denuded epithelium will be visible as a brilliant green.

Rose bengal is a red dye that has an affinity for degenerated epithelium. Similar to fluorescein, it will stain areas in which the epithelium has been sloughed off. However, unlike fluorescein, intact, nonviable epithelial cells of the conjunctiva or cornea will stain brightly with rose bengal. The stain is helpful in diagnosing keratoconjunctivitis sicca or other conditions associated with dryness of the conjunctiva. If the dye stains devitalized epithelium of the nasal bulbar conjunctiva, a diagnosis of keratitis sicca may be made.

EXAMINATION OF THE IRIS

The iris is quite clear for inspection (Fig. 3-12). Generally, both irises are of the same color, but there are individual variations. Color depends on the amount of pigment in the stroma and posterior layer of the iris. A heavily pigmented iris appears brown, whereas a lightly pigmented one appears blue. Interestingly enough, there is not any blue pigment in the iris. In the blue iris, the light passes through the nonpigmented stroma and strikes the pigmented epithelial cells on the back of the iris so that light of

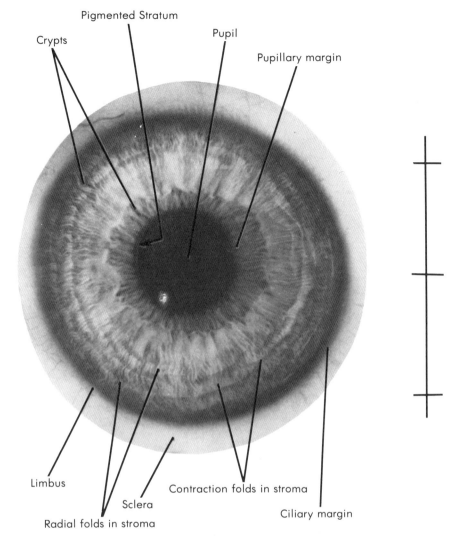

Crypts

Pigmented Stratum

Pupil

Pupillary margin

Limbus

Sclera

Radial folds in stroma

Contraction folds in stroma

Ciliary margin

Fig. 3-12 Anatomy of the iris. (Courtesy Eastman Kodak Company, Rochester, NY.)

longer wavelength (red) is absorbed and that of the shorter wavelength (blue) is reflected.

A difference in the color between the two irises (heterochromia) may indicate a congenital abnormality, iris tumor, retained metallic intraocular foreign body (siderosis), or old iritis.

The iris is normally well supported by the underlying lens. Tremulousness of the iris (iridodenesis) usually means the presence of a dislocated lens. This tremor of the iris is best seen by having the patient look quickly from one point of fixation to another.

A defect in the iris is called a *coloboma*, which indicates absence of some portion of the iris. This may be the result of surgery or may be a congenital abnormality.

EXAMINATION OF THE PUPIL—PUPILLARY REFLEXES

A small penlight is sufficient for examination of the pupillary function. To assess the direct light reflex, the patient should be seated in a dimly illuminated room with the light evenly distributed throughout the room. A small penlight is brought from the side and shone directly into the pupil of one eye. This direct light causes a constriction of the pupil on that side.

To assess the consensual light reflex, the examiner directs the light into one eye while observing the fellow eye. An intact consensual response to light causes constric-

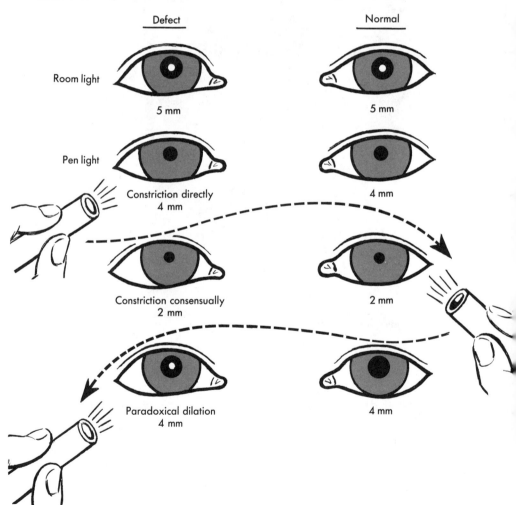

Fig. 3-13 Swinging flashlight test.

tion of the pupil of the unilluminated eye. The swinging flashlight test compares the direct and consensual reflexes in the same eye and is used to determine the absence or presence of an afferent pupillary defect. Bright light is directed on one eye while the response is watched. The light is then swung over to the fellow eye, and the initial reflex to constrict is noted. Under normal conditions, miosis occurs bilaterally as the light is swung back and forth. If conduction is impaired in one eye, the impaired eye will show paradoxical dilation when the light is returned to that eye. This finding is that of an afferent pupillary defect or the Marcus Gunn pupil (Fig. 3-13). The differential diagnosis includes a retinal detachment, occlusion of the central retinal artery or vein, optic neuritis, or optic atrophy.

Differential diagnosis of a dilated pupil

A dilated pupil may be caused by third nerve palsy, trauma, Adie's pupil, or acute glaucoma or may be drug induced.

Third nerve palsy. If the dilated pupil is fixed, the cause may be third nerve palsy. This condition may be associated with ptosis and a motility disturbance, characterized by the eye being deviated out and down. The pupil responds to constricting drops, such as pilocarpine. This is a neurosurgical emergency, and the possibility of an intracranial mass lesion must be ruled out.

Trauma. Damage to the iris sphincter may result from a blunt or penetrating injury. Iris transillumination defects may be visible with the ophthalmoscope or slitlamp, and the pupil may have an irregular shape.

Adie's pupil. In Adie's pupil, the pupil responds better to near stimulation than to light. The condition is thought to be related to aberrant innervation of the iris by axons that normally stimulate the ciliary body. Absent knee jerks is usually associated

Acute glaucoma. The patient may complain of pain and/or nausea and vomiting. The eye is red, vision is diminished, intraocular pressure is elevated, and the pupil is mid-dilated and poorly reactive.

Drug-induced dilation. Iatrogenic or self-contamination may occur with a variety of dilating drops, such as cyclopentolate HCl (Cyclogyl), tropacamide (Mydriacyl), homatropine, scopalamine, and atropine. The pupil is fixed and dilated and, unlike in third nerve palsy, does not respond to constricting drops.

Differential diagnosis of a constricted pupil

A constricted pupil occurs in Horner's syndrome or iritis and may be drug induced.

Horner's syndrome. Other signs of Horner's syndrome include mild ptosis of the upper lid and retraction of the lower lid. The difference in pupillary size is more notable in dim light, since adrenergic innervation to the iris dilator muscle is diminished.

Iritis. Slitlamp examination shows keratic precipitates and cells in the anterior chamber, and there is a prominent ciliary flush. The intraocular inflammation stimulates pupillary constriction.

Drug-induced constriction. Iatrogenic or self-induced pupillary constriction may be

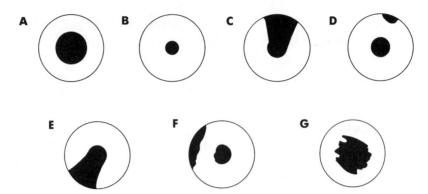

Fig. 3-14 Variations in pupillary size and shape. **A,** Dilated, or mydriatic, pupil. **B,** Constricted, or miotic, pupil. **C,** Full, or sector, iridectomy. **D,** Peripheral iridectomy. **E,** Congenital coloboma of the iris. **F,** Iridodialysis. **G,** Posterior synechiae.

caused by a variety of drugs, including pilocarpine, carbachol, and echothiophate iodide (Phospholine iodide).

Shape. The pupil is normally round and regular. Irregularities of the pupil may result from congenital abnormalities, inflammation of the iris, trauma to the eye, and surgical intervention (Fig. 3-14). Trauma may cause tears of the iris in the form of a wedge-shaped defect, either of the pupillary margin or at its base (iridodialysis). An iris may be bound down to the lens by adhesions (posterior synechiae), and irregular changes may occur in the shape of the pupil.

Equality of size. Pupils should be equal in size and react equally to direct light stimulation, consensual light stimulation, and approaching near objects. In ordinary room light, the diameter of the normal adult pupil is between 3 and 5 mm. If the two pupils are unequal in size, the condition is called anisocoria. The inequality of size may be caused by a tonic pupil (Adie's syndrome). In this condition, which can be mistaken for a partial third nerve palsy, the pupil responds to light stimulation very slowly. Adie's syndrome is diagnosed by the instillation of 2.5% fresh methacholine solution (Mecholyl) into the affected eye, which causes constriction of the tonic pupil, but not of the normal pupil.

Disorders of pupillary function may involve many of the above factors together. For example, the patient with Argyll Robertson pupils, one of the classic signs of late syphilis, has pupils that are small, irregular in shape, and nonreactive to either direct or consensual light stimulation but reactive to near stimulation.

EXAMINATION OF THE ANTERIOR CHAMBER AND ANGLE STRUCTURES

By shining a penlight from the side, one can estimate the depth of the anterior chamber. If the anterior chamber is shallow, it should be so recorded because of the potential danger of narrow-angle glaucoma. Normally the angle structure of the eye is inaccessible for direct illumination. However, with the use of a goniolens applied to the cornea, one can bounce light obliquely through a prism or mirror and view the angle structures of the eye. This lens is of value in determining whether the angle between the cornea and iris is closed or open. It is also useful in determining drainage sites for glaucoma surgery and for evaluating the cause of failure after glaucoma surgery. The mirror type or prism type of goniolens deflects a beam of light into the opposite angle of the anterior chamber. This image is viewed through the slitlamp biomicroscope.

EXAMINATION OF THE OCULAR MUSCLES—STRABISMUS

There are six extraocular muscles in each eye that are innervated by a total of three nerves. The action of specific muscles can vary, depending on the position of the eye when it is innervated. Table 3-2 shows the general relationships that apply.

The examiner should determine the range of ocular movements in all gaze positions (Fig. 3-15). Limited movement in any gaze position can be documented as −1 minimal, −2 moderate, −3 severe, or −4 total. For example, a patient with right sixth nerve palsy can be recorded as shown in Fig. 3-15, B. Fig. 3-15, C shows a record of a blowout fracture to the right orbit with entrapment of the inferior rectus muscle and limitation of upward gaze. Fig. 3-16 illustrates the positions of gaze that may demonstrate weakness of an extraocular muscle.

Alternate cover test

The cover test is perhaps the most widely employed for the detection and measurement of strabismus, tropia, or phoria. It is reliable, easy to perform, and requires no special equipment. The test is conventionally employed at both distance and near, with and without glasses, the eye being examined in the primary position. To ensure fixation in very young children, the fixation object should be an interesting as well as a detailed article, such as a brightly colored toy. Once the examiner is sure that the child is looking at the fixation object, an occluder is interposed in front of one eye. If the left eye is occluded, the following possibilities may ensue:

1. The right eye, which is deviating, may move horizontally (esotropia = moves inward, or exotropia = moves outward), or vertically (hypertropia = moves up,

---

Table 3-2   Extraocular muscle innervation

Innervation	Muscle	Primary action
3rd nerve	Superior rectus	Up and out
3rd nerve	Medial rectus	In
3rd nerve	Inferior rectus	Down and out
3rd nerve	Inferior oblique	Up and in
4th nerve	Superior oblique	Down and in
6th nerve	Lateral rectus	Out

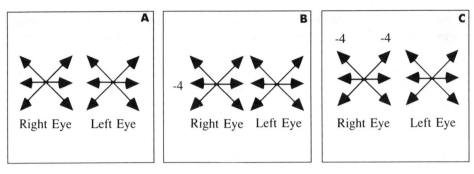

Fig. 3-15   A, Method for examining and recording ocular motility. **B,** Record of a sixth nerve palsy of the right eye. **C,** Record of a right orbital blowout fracture and limited upgaze.

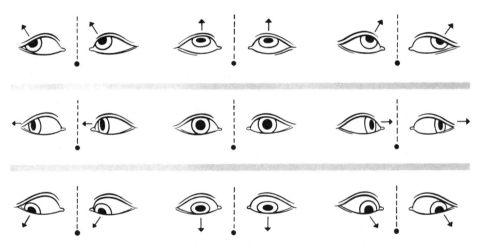

Fig. 3-16   Eye rotations: the primary and eight cardinal positions of gaze that should be tested to detect weakness of an extraocular muscle.

or hypotropia = moves downward), indicating that the child has a manifest strabismus.

2. The right eye may wander slightly, indicating that the fixation of the eye is defective or absent, as may occur with gross amblyopia.

3. There may be no movement of the right eye, indicating that this eye is straight. The procedure is then repeated, this time covering the right eye without allowing the patient to become binocular during testing. Manifest strabismus is revealed by observation of any eye movement of the uncovered eye to take up fixation when the occluder is placed before the fellow eye. Occasionally, a child may be referred who appears to have an ocular deviation, but there is no detectable strabismus. This condition is called pseu-

dostrabismus. In most instances, the appearance is caused by the presence of prominent epicanthal folds that extend from the upper lid, cover the inner canthal region, and blend into the medial aspects of the lower lid. This is a false impression of a turn, more noticeable when the child turns the eye to either side.

OPHTHALMOSCOPY

There are two types of ophthalmoscopes, direct and indirect. By and large, the indirect ophthalmoscope is used by ophthalmologists and permits binocular vision with depth perception (stereoscopic vision). It also permits a wider field of view of a given area.

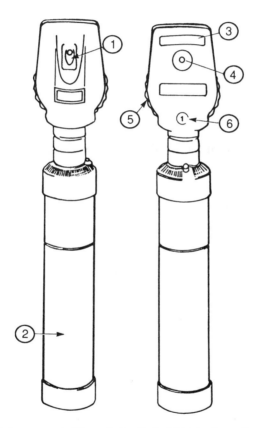

Fig. 3-17   The ophthalmoscope. *1*, Mirror that reflects light into the patient's eye with a viewing hole above, through which the examiner looks. It is in this viewing hole that poitive or negative lenses can be superimposed to adjust focus. *2*, Handle where battery power is supplied. On top of the handle base is a rheostat for light adjustment. *3*, Headrest bar, which goes against the examiner's forehead. *4*, Viewing hole through which the examiner looks. It is this hole that lenses may superimpose for focus. *5*, focusing wheel. While holding the ophthalmoscope, one's index finger can move this wheel to adjuist the lenses in the hole at *4*. *6*, As the dial wheel (*5*) is moved, the power of the lens is indicated in this small window.   (From Coles WH: Ophthalmology: a diagnostic text, Williams & Wilkins, 1989, p. 382.)

The image is inverted. It may be used in the operating room without contamination and permits indentation of the sclera and a better view of the periphery of the fundus. It provides more intense illumination and frees the hands for operative manipulation.

However, the direct ophthalmoscope is the one most popular for all practitioners (Fig. 3-17). This permits a greater magnification ($\times 15$). It is easier to use with small or undilated pupils and is mechanically easier to employ. This ophthalmoscope was popularized more than 100 years ago by Von Helmholtz. The ophthalmoscope contains a number of spherical lenses that aid the practitioner to focus. However, there are no cylindrical lenses, so that if the individual has an astigmatic error of refraction, it cannot be compensated for. The direct ophthalmoscope enables the examiner to use the power of the subject's eyes as a magnifying system to see the retina as an erect picture.

The ophthalmoscope, invented by Von Helmholtz in 1851, permitted analysis of the interior of the eye during life. For the first time, this allowed recognition of changes in the eye grounds, providing valuable information in the diagnosis of disease of the general system as well as of the eye itself.

Ophthalmoscopy is best performed in a dimly lit room to facilitate pupillary dilation. However, for better inspection of the fundus, the pupil should be dilated with a mydriatic agent such as 2.5% phenylephrine (Table 3-3). This does not inhibit accommodation. With heavy pigmented irides, a stronger mydriatic agent will be required.

Table 3-3   Drops used in refraction

Drug	Onset of maximum cycloplegia	Duration of activity	Comment
Atropine sulfate 1%	6-24 hr	10-15 days, especially in a blue-eyed child	Not used routinely except for the assessment of accommodative strabismus in children
Scopolamine hydrobromide 1/4%	30-60 min	3-4 days	Used in atropine-allergic patients
Homatropine hydrobromide 1.25% to 5%	1 hr	1-2 days	Requires an hour to take effect and lasts 2 days; not used routinely
Cyclopentolate hydrochloride 1% (Cyclogyl)	10-45 min	12-24 hr	Active in 20-45 minutes; two sets of drops given 5 minutes apart; a good rapid-acting cycloplegic drop for office use
Tropicamide (Mydriacyl) 0.5%	20-30 min	4-10 hr	A good drug for office use with an effect similar to Cyclogyl
Phenylephrine 2.5% (Neosynephrine)	20-30 min (no cycloplegia)	30 min-2 hr	Does not affect accommodation; helpful in presbyopia for fundus examination

Drops such as cyclopentolate (Cyclogyl 1%) or tropicamide (Midriacyl) should be instilled. These drops do affect accommodation. When inserting a mydriatic cycloplegic drop, one should be sure that the chamber angles are deep. If not, angle closure glaucoma may be induced.

The examiner stands directly in front of the patient and examines the patient's right eye with the examiner's own right eye and the left eye in a similar fashion, with the examiner's left eye. This permits the examiner to be closer to the patient. Both of the examiner's eyes are kept open. The patient is asked to look at the opposite wall over the shoulder of the examiner. The cornea, anterior chamber, and lens structures are first carefully examined at a distance so that one can explore all the medium. Usually the distance is about 15 inches between the patient and the examiner. One gradually approaches the eye of the patient until a red reflex appears. During this period, one will carefully note the cornea, anterior chamber, and lens structures. One then observes a red reflex. This red reflex is a combination of the reflex from the choroidal vasculature and the pigment epithelium. For purposes of orientation, the optic disc is first identified. The color and shape are noted. The disc is an oval structure that represents the site of entrance of the optic nerve (Fig. 3-18). It is usually light pink and may have a central yellowish-white depression called the physiological cup created by a separation of the nerve fibers. The depression may be large and occupy up to half of the disc. At

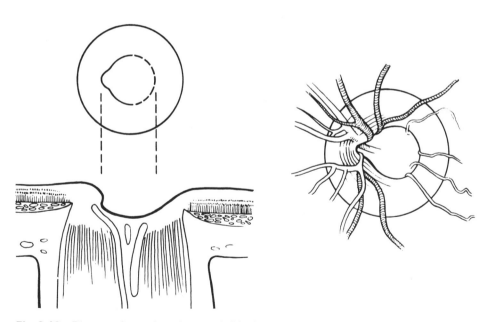

Fig. 3-18 Diagram of a moderately cupped disk viewed on end and in profile, with an accompanying sketch for the patient's record. The width of the central cup divided by the width of the disk is the "cup-to-disk ratio." The cup-to-disk ratio of this disk is approximately 0.5. (From Vaughan D and Asbury T: General ophthalmology, ed. 12, Appleton Lange, 1989, p. 35.)

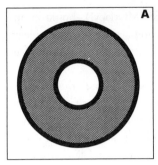 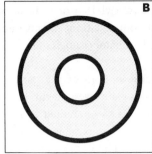 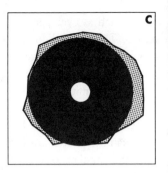

Fig. 3-19   A, The normal neural rim is pink. **B,** The neural rim is pale in an old ischemic optic neuropathy. **C,** Hyperemia of the disc and indistinct disc margins may occur in papilledema, optic neuritis, or ischemic optic neuropathy.

the base of the cup are grayish spots representing the opening of the lamina cribrosa, the connective tissue layer through which the fibers of the optic nerve pass. The cup size is noted, and the margins of the disc are observed. The margins of the disc are sharp and distinct, except for the margins of the upper and lower poles, which may be slightly fuzzy (Fig. 3-19). The blood vessels are then examined. From the disc, the retinal arterioles and veins emerge and bifurcate and extend toward the four quadrants of the retina. The central retinal vein, which is usually found lateral to the central retinal artery, is larger and darker red. The examiner observes for venous pulsation. If venous pulsation is present, it suggests there is no papilledema, because this disappears early. These branch into retinal vesicules and arterioles. The retinoles are darker in color. Retinoles and arterioles will cross over under each other, but an arteriole will never cross over an arteriole, nor would a retinole ever cross a retinole. Approximately two disc diameters away from the optic disc and slightly below (about 1 mm) its center is the macula, about 5.5 mm in diameter. The macula is a small avascular area that appears darker red than the surrounding fundus. At the center of the macula, there is a glistening oval reflex called the *fovea.* At its center is the foveola, which has no rod but a high density of cones. This area is a vascular capillary-free zone. This saves the foveola from vessels that obscure visual acuity. Underlying choriocapillaries supply this capillary-free zone. Cilioretinal arteries arising from the ciliary circulation are seen in about 20% of patients and account for the blood supply to the macular region in these individuals. This is an important fact when occlusion of the central retinal artery occurs, in which the cilioretinal artery provides continual nourishment to the macular region and maintains central acuity. In young people, a second reflex, which appears as a glimmering halo, may surround the entire macular region. Each quadrant of the fundus is examined in turn. For the examiner to see as much of the peripheral retina as possible, the patient should be asked to look in the direction of the quadrant under study. The examiner follows out the arterioles in that particular quadrant to the extreme limit. The color of the fundus is usually an even red hue, but it will vary with the general pigmentation of the underlying choroid and the general pigmentation of the individual. The background is bright orange-red in persons of fair complexion, whereas it is deeper brick red in darker individuals. Some details of the choroidal vessels may be seen in fair individuals and in the periphery.

Most ophthalmoscopes have two or more beam lights of different sizes. The smaller beam light is particularly useful for viewing the fundus through small pupils such as those found in glaucoma patients under treatment with pilocarpine. It eliminates some of the glare around the pupil from reflex scattering from the iris. Cobalt blue filters may be present as an aperture disc in the ophthalmoscope. These are used for fluorescein studies of the fundus as well as examination of the cornea with fluorescein strip papers. Ophthalmoscopes sometimes contain a target so the patient can fixate on the center of the grid for viewing the macular area.

Tips on ophthalmoscopy

1. If the examiner has any significant astigmatic error, he or she should wear corrective glasses.
2. A smaller light spot should be used.
3. The cornea and anterior structures of the eye should be examined from a distance of 1 foot through the sight aperture of the ophthalmoscope. The examiner then moves to within 1 inch of the eye to observe the retina.
4. The patient should be asked to gaze on all quadrants to observe the peripheral retina. Each arteriole is followed out out to the periphery.
5. To avoid coming too close to the patient's eye, the examiner may put his or her middle finger forward and rest it against the patient's cheek. This will provide a proprioceptive method of determining how close the examiner is to the patient.

USE OF THE RETINOSCOPE AND ITS FUNCTION

The retinoscope is a valuable instrument for determining the refractive error in an eye. It is useful in determining the total objective refractive area and may be the only means of assessing refractive error in infants, small children, illiterates, mentally retarded persons, and debilitated or uncooperative individuals.

There are two types of retinoscopes: the spot retinoscope and the streak retinoscope. In both of these instruments, light is reflected from a mirror directly into the pupil and an area of the retina is illuminated. The refractionist sees this as a red reflected reflex glow (Figs. 3-20 and 3-21). In an eye with no refractive error, the rays of light come to a focus on a point on the retina, and the refractionist sees the whole pupil lit with a red glow. If the patient is myopic, the rays of light from the retinoscope come to a focus in front of the retina, cross at this point, and illuminate a relatively large area of the retina behind the focal point. If the light source is moved across the pupil, the rays of light from the retinoscope pivoting on the focal point will move the illuminated area of the fundus in an opposite direction to that of the retinoscope. This apparent shift of the illuminated area is called an *against motion*. The refractionist then

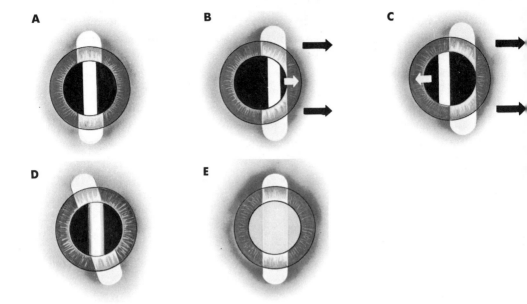

Fig. 3-20 Reflexes produced by the streak retinoscope. **A,** Normal. **B,** "With" movement. The reflex moves in the same direction as the retinoscope, indicating a hyperopic eye. **C,** "Against" movement. The reflex moves in the opposite direction to that of the retinoscope, indicating a myopic eye. **D,** Streak is not uniform in size, speed, or brightness over the entire aperture. The band is more prominent in one meridian, indicating astigmatism. **E,** Neutralization point. There is no movement of the reflex, and the pupil is filled with a red glow.

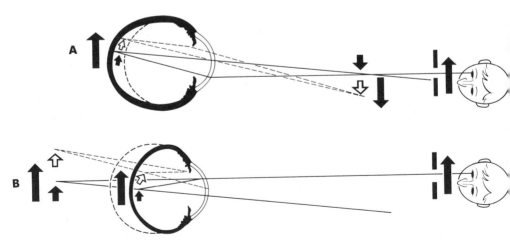

Fig. 3-21 Movement of images on retinoscopy. **A,** Myopia: real upside down image creating against motion. **B,** Hyperopia: virtual upright image creating with motion.

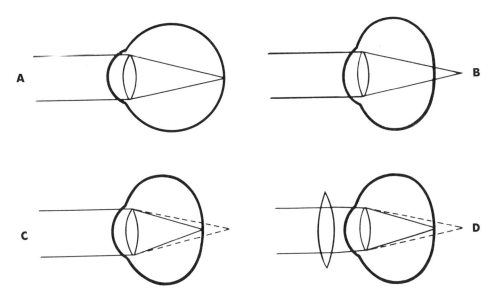

Fig. 3-22 **A,** Emmetropic eye. Parallel rays of light come to a focus on the retina. **B,** Hyperopic eye. Parallel rays of light come to a focus behind the retina in the unaccommodative eye. **C,** Latent hyperopia. Accommodation by the lens of the eye brings parallel rays of light to focus on the retina. **D,** Absolute hyperopia. A convex lens is required to bring rays of light to focus on the retina.

adds minus lenses before the patient's eyes to move the focal point back onto the retina and, when the correct combination of lenses is achieved, the movement of light across the pupil causes no movement of the reflex; it merely turns on and off and lights up the pupil. Conversely, if the patient is hyperopic, the ray of light from the retinoscope on passing through the eye will focus at a point behind the retina (Fig. 3-22). The lateral movement of the retinoscope across the pupil will cause the area illuminated on the retina (that is pivoting on the focal point) to move in the same direction as the retinoscope, indicating that the eye is hyperopic, or far-sighted. This shift is called a *with motion*. The refractionist then adds plus lenses to bring the focussing point up to the retina, until he or she gets the on and off light reflex on the pupil without any apparent movement. If the eye is astigmatic, it will exhibit two powers on axes at 90 degrees to one another (Fig 3-23). The retinoscope is used to correct the power in one axis and then on the opposite axis. In this manner a cylindrical prescription can be obtained. While the retinoscope is an ophthalmologic tool, it can be mastered with practice on schematic eyes as well as eyes with well-dilated pupils.

VISUAL FIELD TESTING

Testing the visual field is a method of stimulating the peripheral retina with test objects to determine perception. Sophisticated visual field equipment is available that maps out the central and peripheral field of vision of each eye. This equipment is usually housed

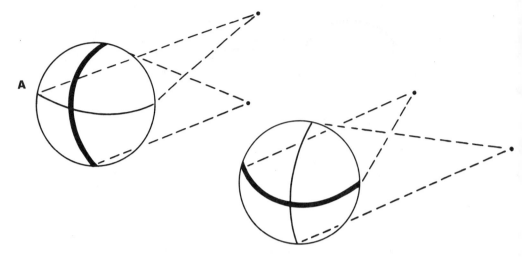

Fig. 3-23 A, Astigmatism with the rule. The vertical corneal meridian has the steepest curvature. **B,** Astigmatism against the rule. The horizontal meridian has the steepest curvature.

in ophthalmologists' offices or university departments and gives a clear picture of whether the peripheral field and central field is intact or whether there has been some field loss. For the purpose of this text, we will confine ourselves to confrontation fields, which is the most widely used because it requires no special facilities or equipment and can be performed on patients in homes, offices, on bedridden patients and in hospitals.

In confrontation testing, the examiner tests the range of the patient's field by that of the examiner's own, which may be considered normal. The examiner stands facing the patient at a distance of approximately 2 feet. Opposite eyes are occluded, that is, the patient's left eye is covered while the examiner closes his or her right eye. Each of them fixes on the exposed eye of the other. The examiner moves a finger or a white test object (for example, a small white hat pin), mounted on a handle such as a pencil from the extreme periphery and notes when it comes into the field of view; the patient and examiner should see it simultaneously (Fig. 3-24). The test is performed while the patient has his back to the light and the background to the examiner is uniform and dark. All four quadrants of the visual fields should be tested and at least two different approaches should be used in each quadrant. If any defect is indicated or suspected from this method, the field should be accurately mapped out and recorded by a more sophisticated method or with a tangent screen.

If vision is extremely poor, a small penlight may be used for a rough test. A modification of this test is to have the patient count fingers in each quadrant. While one eye is occluded, the examiner brings in from the periphery one, two, or three fingers and asks the patient to count the number of fingers brought in from each quadrant. The confrontation field is an excellent method of screening patients and, if used skillfully,

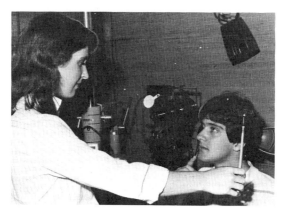

Fig. 3-24 Confrontation test. A test object is brought in from the periphery to the seeing area.

can be surprisingly accurate. It may be the only method of examining children, illiterates, and mentally deficient patients. With children, small articles of interest, such as a brightly colored plastic toy, may be used as a test object. The preservation of the field particularly is indicated when the child makes a quick glance at the object of interest detected in the peripheral field.

However, failure to demonstrate a field defect by confrontation does not imply a normal field. Defects may be present and may be detected by more sophisticated visual field tests. It may be of interest to plot out one's own blind spot along with that of the patient. This can be easily performed by bringing the small pin into the blind spot from the periphery until the pin disappears to both examiner and patient and then noting its re-entrance into the visual field. It should be approximately the same for both the practitioner and the patient if the bead is midway. This blind spot corresponds with the entrance of the optic nerve to the posterior pole of the eye. It is located about 12 to 15 degrees to the outside of the fixation point and about 1.5 degrees below the horizontal meridian. It measures approximately 7.5 degrees in height and 5.5 degrees in width.

A visual field defect may be caused by disturbance of any of the neurologic pathways for light transmission. This includes the retina, optic disc, optic nerve, optic chiasm, optic tract, optic radiations, or occipital cortex.

A normal response should be recorded as shown in Fig. 3-25, A. The patient with a retinal detachment of the superior retina would have an inferior field defect (Fig. 3-25, B). A patient with a pituitary tumor may have a visual loss and a complete bitemporal defect (Fig. 3-25, C). However, as noted before, a more detailed evaluation of the visual field requires more sophisticated equipment. The target size and luminosity may be varied and the patient's response documented on a computer-generated printout of the visual field. Errors in visual fields may occur if vision is degraded by such media opacities as corneal scars or cataracts. Larger test objects may be required.

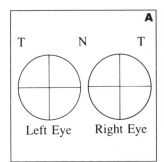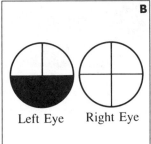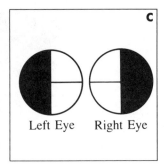

Fig. 3-25 **A,** A normal gross visual field test. (T = Temporal field; N = Nasal field. **B,** An inferior field defect of the left eye; the right eye is normal. **C,** A complete bitemporal visual field defect.

MEASUREMENT OF INTRAOCULAR PRESSURE
Principles of Schiøtz and applanation tonometry

The most important reason for checking intraocular pressure is to rule out raised intraocular pressure. This may occur in acute-angle closure glaucoma, which is a painful condition and in which the intraocular pressure is greater than 40 mm. However, wide-angle glaucoma may exist that is not accompanied by any symptoms or signs until late in the disease. It is usually detected by a raised intraocular pressure. A pressure over 22 mm Hg is generally considered above average and should prompt further investigation.

Glaucoma affects an estimated 2% of adults over the age of 40; in fact, some authors have found elevated intraocular pressure (greater than 22 mm Hg) among as many as 4.7% to 6.5% of normal individuals. The incidence is higher in the elderly.

A number of methods are used to check intraocular pressure. The two basic methods are Schiøtz tonometry and applanation tonometry. (Fig. 3-26). Airpuff tonometry is a form of applanation tonometer in which there is no contact with the eye; a puff of air comes out of a sophisticated machine that in turn flattens the cornea and reads out the amount of pressure. Applanation tonometry requires sophisticated equipment and an attachment to a slitlamp biomicroscope. It takes more experience to master but results in a more accurate measurement. This is expensive and beyond the scope of this text for the beginner practitioner for which the book is intended. A detailed account of applauation tonometry may be found in the text, *The Ophthalmic Assistant*. Following are comparisons between the Schiøtz tonometer and the applanation tonometer:

1. The Schiøtz tonometer indents the cornea, whereas the applanation tonometer flattens it (Fig. 3-27).
2. The Schiøtz tonometer is portable; the conventional applanation tonometer is not. There are, however, some portable applanation tonometers.
3. The Schiøtz tonometer measures the amount of corneal indentation produced by a given weight (Fig. 3-28). The applanation tonometer measures the amount of force required to produce a constant corneal flattening.

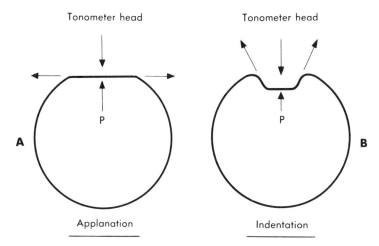

Tonometer head   Tonometer head

P   P

A   B

Applanation   Indentation

Fig. 3-26 Comparison of applanation and indentation tonometry. **A,** In applanation tonometry the cornea is flattened and the pressure is distributed evenly on each side; the pressure measurement is very close to that of the undisturbed eye. **B,** Indentation of the cornea causes buckling of the ocular coats because of the oblique distribution of pressure.

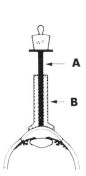

A

B

Fig. 3-27 Principle of the indentation tonometer. **A,** Plunger to indent cornea. **B,** Frame resting on cornea. (From Reinecke R, Stein H, and Slatt B: Introductory manual for the ophthalmic assistant, St Louis, 1972, The CV Mosby Co.)

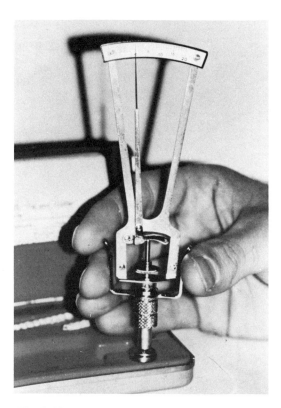

Fig. 3-28 Metallic test plate for Schiøtz tonometer.

4. The Schiøtz tonometer raises the intraocular pressure because of indentation and the weight of the instrument itself. The applanation tonometer exerts only a small force on the cornea.

5. The Schiøtz tonometer may give an inaccurate measure because of the distention of the ocular coats. In high myopia, a condition in which the sclera is usually thin, a false low pressure reading may be obtained. The footplate of the instrument is shaped to the average corneal curvature, but most patients' corneas are not exact fits required by the footplate of the Schiøtz tonometer. This poor fit introduces errors. Readings with the applanation tonometer are relatively independent of the rigidity of the ocular coats and are unaffected by corneal curvature variations.

6. Because of the buckling of the cornea and the resulting displacement of aqueous humor by the Schiøtz tonometer, second and third readings may be slightly lower as a result of massage of aqueous humor out of the eye. This does not occur with the applanation tonometer.

7. The Schiøtz tonometer measures tension with the patient in the recumbent position; the conventional applanation tonometer measures tension with the patient in the sitting position. However, there is a handheld applanation tonometer that can be used with the patient in any position.

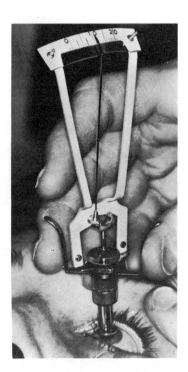

Fig. 3-29 Measurement of intraocular pressure with the Schiøtz tonometer. Note that the lids are pinioned against the bony orbit by the examiner's fingers.

How to perform Schiøtz tonometry

The patient is usually placed in a recumbent position, with his head tilted backward, and is asked to look up at a fixation point directly vertical above him (Fig. 3-29). If he is not able to see well, his thumb may be placed in front of his fellow eye so that he may visualize his thumb. The corneas are anesthetized with topical anesthetic such as proparacaine (Ophthaine) or pontocaine. If the blinking motion is excessive, the examiner may pinion the lid against the margin of the orbit with his or her fingers, taking care not to press on the globe itself. The tonometer head is allowed to rest on the patient's cornea. The extent to which the plunger of the tonometer indents the cornea is in effect the measurement of its intraocular pressure. The greater the distance the plunger indents the cornea, the softer the eye and the lower the intraocular pressure. This is recorded on the scale of the tonometer, where the scale reading reflects the excursion distance of the plunger. If the eye is soft, as the Schiøtz tonometer plunger moves, the recording needle moves further along the scale. The higher the scale reading, the lower the eye pressure. Conversely, minimal excursion of the plunger suggests that the eye is firm and the intraocular pressure high. If this occurs, additional weights may be required until the cornea is indented and the scale reads over 3. The indicator on the tonometer points to the scale readings of the tonometer. Converting from scale readings with Schiotz tonometry to millimeters of mercury requires a conversion table or graph (Table 3-4). This is usually supplied with the instrument. This chart converts plunger excursion into intraocular pressure of millimeters of mercury.

Cleansing of the tonometer

The necessity for sterility of the tonometer itself is controversial. Many ophthalmologists do nothing regarding the sterility of the base of the tonometer, except to make sure that it is not placed on an infectious eye. Others use an alcohol lamp and flame at the base. Some ophthalmologists house the tonometer in an ultraviolet sterilizer.

Since the AIDS problem has surfaced, however, hydrogen peroxide has come to be used in some practices because it is an excellent disinfectant. It should be remembered that the AIDS virus has been isolated from tear secretions. A disposable rubber cap, the Tonofilm, fits over the base of the tonometer and is an excellent device for maintaining sterility between patients.

Aids in good tonometry (Schiøtz tonometry)

1. The instrument should be kept clean so that the plunger moves freely. All the parts should be disassembled and the barrel of the tonometer freed of mucous deposits by using a pipe cleaner or a brush moistened with alcohol. This cleaning routine should be performed daily.
2. A system for sterilization should be developed.
3. The instrument should measure zero when resting on the curved metal block provided with each instrument.
4. Scale readings of 3 or less are not reliable. If the scale reading is too low, a higher

Table 3-4   1955 calibration scale for Schiøtz tonometers*

Tonometer reading	Pressure (mm Hg)			
	5.5 g	**7.5 g**	**10 g**	**15 g**
0.0	41.5	59.1	81.7	127.5
0.5	37.8	54.2	75.1	117.9
1.0	34.5	49.8	69.3	109.3
1.5	31.6	45.8	64.0	101.4
2.0	29.0	42.1	59.1	94.3
2.5	26.6	38.8	54.7	88.0
3.0	24.4	35.8	50.6	81.8
3.5	22.4	33.0	46.9	76.2
4.0	20.6	30.4	43.4	71.0
4.5	18.9	28.0	40.2	66.2
5.0	17.3	25.8	37.2	61.8
5.5	15.9	23.8	34.4	57.6
6.0	14.6	21.9	31.8	53.6
6.5	13.4	20.1	29.4	49.9
7.0	12.2	18.5	27.2	46.5
7.5	11.2	17.0	25.1	43.2
8.0	10.2	15.6	23.1	40.2
8.5	9.4	14.3	21.3	38.1
9.0	8.5	13.1	19.6	34.6
9.5	7.8	12.0	18.0	32.0
10.0	7.1	10.9	16.5	29.6
10.5	6.5	10.0	15.1	27.4
11.0	5.9	9.0	13.8	25.3
11.5	5.3	8.3	12.6	23.3
12.0	4.9	7.5	11.5	21.4
12.5	4.4	6.8	10.5	19.7
13.0	4.0	6.2	9.5	18.1
13.5		5.6	8.6	16.5
14.0		5.0	7.8	15.1
14.5		4.5	7.1	13.7
15.0		4.0	6.4	12.6
15.5			5.8	11.4
16.0			5.2	10.4
16.5			4.7	9.4
17.0			4.2	8.5
17.5				7.7
18.0				6.9
18.5				6.2
19.0				5.6
19.5				4.9
20.0				4.5

*Approved by the Committee on Standardization of Tonometers of the American Academy of Ophthalmology and Otolaryngology.

weight should be used. The commonly used weights are 5.5 g, 7.5 g, and 10 g. It should be noted that the lower the scale reading, the higher the pressure in terms of millimeters of mercury.

5. The patient should be comfortable, well anesthetized with drops, and relaxed. Fixation should be maintained on one spot. The most common error in Schiøtz tonometry results from the patient's squeezing the lids together, thus either preventing the easy application of the tonometer to the cornea or gripping it like a vice. The lids must be manually opened by the examiner without any pressure on the globe.

6. The fingers of the examiner must never press on the globe at any time. This extraneous pressure will cause absurd elevations in the intraocular pressure. The tonometer must be applied directly over the apex of the cornea and not be allowed to slide over the surface of the cornea. This may result in corneal abrasions as well as producing errors in measurement.

7. If possible, tonometry should be avoided on an infected eye as a prevention against spread of the infectious organisms from eye to eye or patient to patient.

8. For inexperienced examiners, practice with the instrument may be performed on someone with an artificial eye. This will eliminate the fear of danger to the patient's or a colleague's eye.

USE OF MAGNIFYING DEVICES

Magnifying devices are employed for partially sighted individuals. A partially sighted individual has vision of 20/60 or worse in the best corrected eye. Included in this classification of the partially sighted are persons who are legally blind—who have a visual acuity of 20/200 or worse in the better eye—or persons with a field restriction of 20 degrees or less. Most of these individuals with subnormal vision can be assisted by properly selected optical aids.

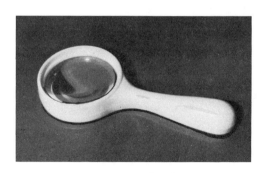

Fig. 3-30 Hand magnifier, ×5.

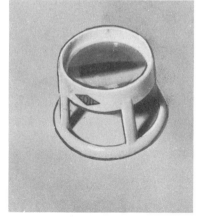

Fig. 3-31 Stand magnifier, ×5.

Optical aids are divided into conventional lenses and magnifying lenses (Figs. 3-30 and 3-31). The degree of magnification required will, of course, depend on the patient's visual acuity and age and the work for which the optical aid is designed. A rule of thumb is devised in terms of visual acuity alone. The numerator of the patient's distant visual acuity is divided into the denominator; the result should be approximately equal to the magnification required for Jaeger 5 (J5) on the near vision chart. This figure is doubled for a lens to achieve J1. For example:

20/100 = +5.00 for J5, +10 for J1

20/200 = +10.00 for J5, +20.00 for J1

20/400 = +20.00 for J5, +40.00 for J1

The use of strong convex lenses between +4.00 and +6.00 diopters is the most popular method today for providing magnification. The strong convex lens has a short focal distance so that the reading material can be brought close to the eye. For example, with spectacles of +5.00 diopters, print is held about 9 inches away, whereas with a +20.00 diopter lens the reading distance is only 2 inches from the spectacle. The closer the print to the eye, the larger the image is on the retina. These lens powers can be incorporated into reading glasses or into the bifocal segment of the glasses.

All magnifying devices function by effectively enlarging the size of the retinal image. A similar effect can be produced by bringing the object closer to the eye, since an object viewed at 10 inches has a retinal image twice the size of the same object viewed at 20 inches. These magnifying devices include hand readers and stand magnifiers. Some are illuminated. There are also projection devices, including movie screens, and television and slide projectors. These are bulky and costly, and they lack portability and versatility.

For viewing distant objects, telescopes or binoculars can be used sometimes. Sawing an opera glass in half, for practical use, is a favorite way for the partially sighted to see (Fig. 3-32). The patient will often have to try different aids to determine which is best.

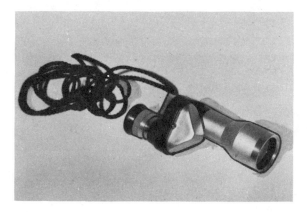

Fig. 3-32 Half of a miniature binocular used as a visual aid.

Examiners may employ optical devices with 2 to 3× magnification during surgery. Usually a second lens is placed in front of the primary lens, as occurs in a Gallilean telescope.

APPLICATION OF AN EYE PATCH

Eye patches are used to immobilize the eyes and protect them from accidental trauma while the eye is healing. Eye patches prevent infection and absorb discharge. Most eye pads have a cotton center and a fine mesh surface to prevent the cotton from being absorbed by the discharge and entering the wound.

An eye pad is secured in place with the application of three or four strips of adhesive or cellophane tape. Strips are directed at an angle from the cheek to the forehead away from the margins of the mouth so that eating will not be hampered and so that when the patient smiles or chews, the bandage will not be loosened significantly.

4 Common eye medications

The clinician should have an understanding of all the commonly used ocular medications. In prescribing eye medications or in seeing patients that are on ocular medications, a knowledge of the mechanisms of action and potential side effects may be valuable. It is well known that certain eye medications have been associated with systemic problems that include myocardial infarction, CNS symptoms, and kidney stones. In addition, specific eye medications can result in ocular complications that include glaucoma, cataracts, ptosis, and keratitis.

MYDRIATIC AND CYCLOPLEGIC AGENTS

Mydriatic drugs dilate the pupil. Cycloplegic agents, in addition to dilating the pupil, act on the ciliary body musculature to inhibit accommodation.

Mydriatic agent

Phenylephrine
- Synthetic sympathomimetic amine primarily used as a mydriatic
- Strength: 0.12, 0.125, 0.2, 2.5, and 10%

Actions
- Mydriasis—produced by stimulation of alpha receptors in the iris dilator muscle; alpha stimulation is overcome by bright light that stimulates a parasympathetic response and results in pupillary constriction
- Decrease ptosis—useful in mild ptosis secondary to Horner's syndrome; the drug stimulates Müller's muscle of the lid and results in a decrease in ptosis

Side effects
Systemic
- Hypertension
- Myocardial infarction

Fifteen cases of acute myocardial infarction were documented (Fraunfelder, 1978) after 10% phenylephrine was instilled. Therefore this drug should be used with great caution in patients with cardiac disease or vascular-occlusive problems.

Table 4-1

	Mydriasis (maximum effect in minutes)	Cycloplegia (maximum effect in hours)	Full recovery (days)
Atropine	40	2-6	10-14
Scopolamine	35	1	7
Homatropine	30	1	1-3
Cyclogyl	25	0.5	1
Tropicamide	20	0.3	0.2

Ocular
- Angle-closure glaucoma
- Pseudoiritis

Liberation of iris pigment granules that mimic aqueous cells. There is no flare that helps to differentiate this from a true iritis.

- Allergy

Mydriatic and cycloplegic agents

Mydriatic and cycloplegic agents (Table 4-1) prevent the acetylcholine effect by reacting with postsynaptic receptors. These drugs paralyze the iris sphincter muscle, which leads to pupillary dilation by the unapposed action of the sympathetic dilator muscle. In addition, these agents will act on the ciliary musculature to inhibit the accommodative effect of the lens, that is, cycloplegia.

Indications
- Dilation of the pupil for funduscopy—short-acting agents are used, such as cyclogyl or tropicamide
- Treatment of iritis—relief of pain by paralyzing the ciliary body; these agents are also used to prevent synechiae, for example, iris-lens adhesions, by dilating the pupil
- Cycloplegic refraction—used in an ophthalmic examination to inhibit accommodation so that the refractive error for glasses or contact lenses can be determined

Side effects
Ocular
- Elevated intraocular pressure—Dilation of the pupil can occasionally precipitate angle-closure glaucoma in a patient with narrow angles
- Impaired accommodation—this may result in a decrease in vision at near and/or distance

Systemic (dry as a bone/red as a beet/mad as a hatter)
- Dry mouth—salivary secretion and gastric secretion impaired
- Flushing—sweating impaired
- Urinary retention
- Tachycardia—caused by vagus block
- CNS symptoms—restlessness, delirium

TOPICAL ANESTHETICS

Topical anesthetics play an important role in ophthalmology. They anesthetize the eye so that intraocular pressure can be checked and minor surgery can be undertaken (for example, removal of a corneal foreign body).

Mechanism of action

- Block action potential of neurons by stabilizing cell membranes
- Cell membranes are stabilized primarily by decreasing sodium conductance (that is, sodium movement into the cell) and to a lesser extent by decreasing potassium conductance out of the cell

Proparacaine (Ophthaine)

- Produces rapid corneal anesthesia when used as a 0.5% solution
- Tonometry can be performed within 20 seconds
- Anesthesia lasts between 10 and 20 minutes
- Burns less than tetracaine

Tetracaine

- Onset and duration of action similar to that of proparacaine
- Major drawback is that it burns significantly

Cocaine

- First drug used as a topical anesthetic; introduced in 1884
- Rapid onset of action; lasts 10 to 20 minutes
- Also acts to dilate the pupil

Indications

- Aid in removal of foreign body
- To make patient more comfortable in traumatic or infected cases so as to allow an adequate examination
- Checking intraocular pressure

Side effects

- Corneal toxicity (more common with cocaine)
- Delayed corneal epithelial healing

Comment

Do not allow patients to use a topical anesthetic outside the office. The anesthetic will impair epithelial healing and prevent resolution of a corneal epithelial defect (for example, abrasion).

ANTIMICROBIALS

The clinician should understand the commonly used topical antibiotic preparations for the eye. Below are the mechanism of action, spectrum of activity, and adverse reactions of the most commonly used ophthalmic antibiotics.

Sulfonamides

Mechanism of action
- Inhibits bacterial folic acid metabolism; bacteriostatic
Spectrum
- Broad spectrum, gram-positive and gram-negative bacteria
Indication
- Useful in conjunctivitis as a drop or ointment
Side effects
- Allergic reaction
- Stevens-Johnson syndrome (rare)

Aminoglycosides (Gentamicin, Tobramycin, Neomycin)

Mechanism of action
- Act on bacterial ribosomes to prevent protein synthesis
Spectrum
- Wide spectrum, especially gram-negative organisms (such as *Pseudomonas, Proteus*)
Indication
- Used topically as a drop or ointment in conjunctivitis
Side effects
- Allergy, especially with neomycin
- Corneal toxicity

Chloramphenicol

Mechanism of action
- Bacteriostatic, reversible binding to bacterial ribosomes and inhibition of protein synthesis
Spectrum
- Broad spectrum, gram-positive and gram-negative; however, resistant to *Pseudomonas*
Indication
- Useful topically as a drop or ointment in conjunctivitis
Side effects
- Aplastic anemia—idiosyncratic bone marrow toxicity; fatal aplastic anemia 1:50,000; four cases of aplastic anemia documented after topical therapy in 3 decades of use
- Dose-related reversible anemia

Erythromycin

Mechanism of action
- Bacteriostatic
Spectrum of activity
- Most gram-positive and some gram-negative bacteria, including *Haemophilus influenzae*

Indication
- Useful as an ointment in staphlycoccal blepharitis
Side effects
- Unusual when given topically

Bacitracin

Mechanism of action
- Bactericidal
Spectrum of activity
- Many gram-positive and some gram-negative bacteria, including *H. influenzae* and *Actinomyces*
Indications
- For conjunctivitis, to be used as a drop or ointment
Adverse effects
- Allergy
- Toxicity

ANTIVIRALS

The ocular viral infections for which there are effective antiviral agents are herpes simplex and herpes zoster. There is no effective agent for adenovirus, the most common cause of viral conjunctivitis. Listed below are the most common antiviral drugs.

Idoxuridine (IDU, Herplex, Stoxil)

Preparation
- Ointment
Mechanism of action
- Competes with thymidine for incorporation into DNA, thereby inhibiting viral DNA synthesis
Spectrum of activity
- Herpes simplex
Adverse reactions
- Epithelial toxicity
- Stenosis or occlusion of lacrimal puncta

Adenine Arabinoside (Vidarabine, Vira-A)

Preparation
- Ointment
Mechanism of action
- Structural analog of nucleic acid that arrests the growth of the viral deoxynucleotide chain, resulting in an ineffective virus
Spectrum of activity
- Herpes simplex

Adverse reactions

- See idoxuridine

Comment

- As effective as idoxuridine in treating herpes simplex keratitis. There is no cross-resistence between adenine arabinoside and idoxuridine. Therefore it is useful in the treatment of herpes simplex strains resistant to idoxuridine or in patients allergic to idoxuridine.

Trifluorothymidine (Trifluridine, Viroptic)

Preparation

- Drop

Mechanism of action

- Competes with thymidine for incorporation into DNA

Spectrum of activity

- Herpes simplex

Adverse reactions

- See idoxuridine

Comment

- Currently the drug of choice for herpes simplex keratitis; has superior corneal penetration than idoxuridine or adenine arabinoside

Acycloguanosine (acyclovir)

Preparation

- Topical (ointment), oral or intravenous

Mechanism of action

- Functions as a substrate for viral thymidine kinase but not for cellular thymidine kinase; acyclovir can enter the sequence of DNA formation only in cells infected by virus

Spectrum of activity

- Herpes simplex and herpes zoster are the main viral indications

Adverse reactions

- Generally uncommon; decreased renal function has been reported with intravenous therapy

Comment

- In herpes zoster ophthalmicus, acycloguanosine at 800 mg po 5×/day for 10 days has been shown to promote more rapid resolution of the skin lesions and decreases the potential ocular complications. The medication should be started early in the disease course, preferably within 48 hours of the onset of the skin lesions.

ANTIFUNGALS

Fungal infections of the eye most commonly involve the cornea as an infiltrate or area of ulceration. Antifungal medications for the eye are usually given in a topical preparation.

Amphotericin-B

Preparation
- Drop, subconjunctival injection, intravenous

Mechanism of action
- Binds to susceptible membranes, results in leakage of essential intracellular constituents

Spectrum
- Useful against candidiasis, sporotrichosis, aspergillosis, cryptococcosis, mucormycosis, histoplasmosis, coccidioidomycosis, blastomycosis, and similar conditions

Miconazole

Preparation
- Drop or ointment

Spectrum
- Broad spectrum antifungal agent

Mechanism of action
- Damages fungal cell walls

Natamycin (Pimaricin)

Preparation
- Drop

Mechanism of action
- Fungacidal effect by damaging fungal cell walls

Spectrum
- Broad spectrum antifungal agent

Comment
- Less irritating to the eye than amphotericin

Ketoconazole

Preparation
- Oral

Mechanism of action
- Increases fungal cell membrane permeability

Spectrum
- Broad spectrum antifungal agent; may also be useful in acanthamoeba keratitis (parasitic infection)

STEROIDS

Corticosteroids are effective antiinflammatory agents with a variety of uses in ophthalmology. The clinician should have a general understanding of the antiinflammatory effects, commonly used agents, ophthalmic indications, and adverse effects of steroids.

Antiinflammatory effects

- Decreases exudation
- Inhibition of fibroblasts and collagen formation
- Retardation of epithelial regeneration
- Decreases neovascularization

Common ocular steroid drops

- Prednisolone acetate 1.0% (Pred Forte)
- Prednisolone phosphate 1.0% (Inflamase Forte)
- Dexamethasone phosphate 0.1% (Decadron)
- Dexamethasone alcohol 0.1% (Maxidex)
- Fluorometholone 0.1% (FML)
- Medrysone (HMS)

Steroid features

- Fluorometholone (FML) and medrysone (HMS) do not penetrate the cornea very well and are mainly used for superficial problems
- Prednisolone and dexamethasone do penetrate the cornea and are effective in problems of the anterior segment of the eye, including iritis
- Acetate preparations penetrate the intact cornea more effectively than phosphate
- Phosphate preparations available as solutions
- Alcohol and acetate preparations available as suspensions; hence must be shaken before use

Indications

- Iritis
- Episcleritis
- Scleritis
- Inflammatory corneal edema
- Postoperatively (for example, after cataract surgery, corneal transplant, or glaucoma procedure)

Adverse ocular effects

- Activation of infections
- Cataracts (posterior subcapsular)
- Glaucoma

GLAUCOMA MEDICATIONS

A variety of medications are used in the management of glaucoma. The most common drugs will be discussed in this section. The clinician should have a general understanding of these medications and be aware of the potential systemic complications.

Beta-adrenergic blockers

Beta-adrenergic blockers are the most common medications used in the initial treatment of open-angle glaucoma. These agents include the beta-1 and beta-2 blockers (Timolol and levobunolol) and beta-1 blockers (eg, Betaxolol).

Timolol (Timoptic) and levobunolol (Betagan)

- Nonselective beta-1 and beta-2 blocking agent
- Decreases aqueous production of the ciliary body
- Onset of action: after 20 minutes
- Maximum reduction of IOP: 1-2 hours
- Duration of action: <24 hours
- No changes in pupil size or accommodation
- As a result of extensive pigment binding of beta-adrenergic antagonists, a residual effect on intraocular pressure can be observed for 2 weeks after discontinuation of therapy
- A pure beta-1 blocker may be of lower risk for patients with chronic obstructive pulmonary disease and peripheral vascular occlusive problems

Adverse effects

Systemic

- Pulmonary: bronchospasm
- Cardiovascular: bradycardia (average decrease 2.9 beats/min); increased heart block; hypotension
- CNS: confusion; hallucinations
- GI: nausea; diarrhea

Ocular

- Corneal anesthesia
- Allergic blepharoconjunctivitis
- Decreased lacrimal secretion

Contraindications

- Cardiovascular disease: congestive heart failure, bradycardia, heart block, hypotension
- Obstructive pulmonary disease: asthma, emphysema, and so on
- Caution in insulin-dependent diabetics, because beta blockers may cause hypoglycemia

Betaxolol (Betoptic)

- Strength 0.5%; frequency: once or twice daily
- Selective beta-1 blocker
- Decreases aqueous secretion as other beta blockers
- By elimination of beta-2 blockade, there are fewer pulmonary side effects

Pilocarpine

- Strength: 0.25% to 10%; frequency: four times daily; drop preparation

- Maximum pressure effect 2 hours after instillation; not related to pupil size
- Iris pigment is a specific binding site for pilocarpine, thus in heavily pigmented eyes the miosis and effect on IOP is reduced
- Also available in a sustained release form; pilocarpine embedded in hydrophilic polymers inserted in the cul-de-sac; one problem is the burst phenomenon, in which there is a large initial release of pilocarpine after insertion, which causes severe miosis and ciliary body spasm; another problem with these devices is the number of patients who have difficulty retaining the device in their cul-de-sac; advantage: maximum duration of pressure control

Action

- Contraction of iris sphincter (miosis)—may be undesirable, especially in patients with cataracts
- Contraction of ciliary muscle (accommodation)—produces miosis; may be disabling in individuals under 50 years of age
- Decreases intraocular pressure as a result of improvement in outflow—contraction of the longitudinal fibers of the ciliary body musculature, which pulls the scleral spur posteriorly, which widens the pores of the trabecular meshwork or opens a collapsed canal of Schlemm

Side effects
Ocular

- Accommodative spasm and pain
- Allergic or toxic reaction
- Pseudodecrease in visual field

Systemic (parasympathetic effects)

- Vomiting
- Diarrhea
- Sweating
- Lacrimation

Carbachol (Isoptocarbachol)

- Strengths 0.75% to 3.0%; frequency: three times daily
- Structurally: combination of portions of physostigmine and acetylcholine molecules; *direct effect* (like pilocarpine) plus *indirect effect* (displacing acetylcholine from the parasympathetic nerve terminals)
- More prolonged action than pilocarpine, and is a more powerful miotic; however, carbachol causes more severe headaches and accommodative spasms of the eye than pilocarpine
- Usually prescribed for patients who are allergic to pilocarpine or whose condition cannot be adequately controlled by pilocarpine
- No systemic effects—unlike pilocarpine

Echothiophate (Phospholine iodide)

- Strength: 0.03%, 0.06%, 0.125%, 0.25%; frequency: twice daily
- Primarily inactivates pseudocholinesterase and secondarily inactivates true cholinesterase
- In glaucoma the 0.06% solution is more effective than 4% pilocarpine and has about the same incidence of patient complaints
  ### Side effects
  ### Ocular
- Accomodative spasm
- Iris cysts—miotic cysts of the pupillary pigment margin; dose related
- Cataracts—anterior subcapsular vacuoles may develop that can progress to anterior subcapsular cataracts; after three years of continuous use, 50% of patients will show decrease visual acuity of 2 lines or more
- Toxic follicular conjunctivitis
  ### Systemic
- Nausea and vomiting, diarrhea, abdominal cramps
- Salivation, sweating, bradycardia
- CNS (hallucinations, depression)
  ### Indications
- Aphakic patients with open-angle glaucoma—cataractogenesis is obviously not of clinical concern
- Esotropia—To medically keep the eyes straight by decreasing the accommodative effect of the muscle imbalance; useful only in specific types of esotropia
- Lice infestations of the lashes—adult form is susceptible, nits are more resistant and must be removed mechanically

Dipivalyl-epinephrine (Propine)

- dipivalyl-epinephrine: increased lipid solubility by 100 to 600× over epinephrine alone; increases corneal penetration by a factor of 17×
- Twice daily dosage provides round-the-clock IOP control
  ### Indications
- Usually glaucoma patients whose condition is not adequately controlled by a beta blocker
- Although not as potent as pilocarpine, Propine is usually preferred in younger patients who are often bothered by pilocarpine-induced accommodative myopia or patients with cataracts because of miosis and a further decrease in vision
  ### Adverse effects
  ### Systemic
- Elevated blood pressure
- Tachycardia
- Headache
- Cerebrovascular accidents

Ocular

- Allergic blepharoconjunctivitis
- Mydriasis
- Cystoid maculopathy (may occur in aphakes)

Carbonic anhydrase inhibitors

- Acetazolamide (Diamox): 125-500 mg; frequency: 1-4 times daily
- Methazolamide (Neptazane): 50-100 mg; frequency: 1-3 times daily
    ### Mechanism of action
- Lower intraocular pressure by reducing aqueous secreation by the ciliary body
    ### Indications
- In the acute management of severely elevated intraocular pressures, for example, acute angle-closure glaucoma, hyphema, postoperative cases
- In the long-term management of glaucoma patients whose pressures cannot be adequately controlled with topical medication
- Pseudotumor cerebri—carbonic anhydrase inhibitors reduce cerebrospinal fluid formation by 20% to 30%
    ### Adverse reactions
    Ocular
- Induced myopia
    Systemic
- Symptom complex of malaise, fatigue, depression, anorexia, weight loss; related to systemic acidosis
- GI distress, characterized by abdominal cramps, burning, irritation, or nausea
- Sulfonamide sensitivity manifested by skin rash
- Aplastic anemia, an idiosyncratic reaction
- Paresthesias commonly affect the hands and feet—manifested as numbness and tingling
- Kidney stones, believed to be a result of calcium precipitation secondary to decrease of citrate and/or magnesium excretion in the urine
    ### Contraindications
- Sulfa allergy
- Kidney disease
- History of stone formation on a carbonic anhydrase inhibitor

5 Commonly seen eye diseases and disorders

This chapter will deal with common diseases and disorders affecting the eye. It will certainly not be comprehensive for the numerous conditions that occasionally or rarely affect the eye.

GLAUCOMA

Glaucoma, from the Greek, *glaukos*, meaning bluish-gray, is a localized ocular disease characterized by (1) elevated intraocular pressure, (2) optic nerve cupping, and (3) visual field loss. The hallmark of glaucoma is an elevated intraocular pressure, which leads to pressure and atrophy of the optic nerve and subsequent loss of the visual field. Glaucoma affects an estimated 2% of adults over the age of 40 years and rises higher in those over 65 years. Glaucoma roughly falls into four classifications:

1 *Primary angle-closure glaucoma.* In this condition there is a sudden marked rise in the intraocular pressure caused by mechanical obstruction of angle structures of the eye at the root of the iris. The vision is lost rapidly, the eye becomes red and the patient complains of excruciating pain (Fig. 5-1), often associated with nausea and vomiting.

2 *Open-angle, or chronic, glaucoma.* The condition is thought to arise from a progressive narrowing of the openings in the trabecular meshwork of the anterior chamber angle structures. The accompanying obstruction to outflow induces a small rise in intraocular pressure. It is insidious and symptomless, initially causing excavation of the optic disc and erosion of the peripheral visual field. Most glaucoma falls into this group.

3 *Secondary glaucoma.* Secondary glaucoma can be of either the open-angle or the narrow-angle type. The elevated intraocular pressure results from some specific disease within the eye, (eg. iritis, tumor, neovascularization), which interferes with aqueous outflow.

4 *Congenital, or infantile, glaucoma.* This condition is often referred to as *buphthalmos* (from Greek *buph*, ox), since the softer infantile eyeball distends as a result of the elevated intraocular pressure and may eventually resemble the large, prominant eye of an ox.

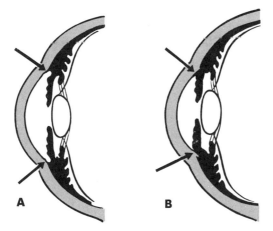

Fig. 5-1 Glaucoma. **A,** Open-angle glaucoma. The obstruction to aqueous flow lies in the trabecular meshwork. **B,** Closed-angle glaucoma. The trabecular meshwork is covered by the root of the iris.

Primary angle-closure glaucoma

Primary angle-closure glaucoma constitutes approximately 30% of all glaucoma. These patients have a shallow anterior chamber and a narrow entrance into the angle. The narrowing is mainly caused by the increased growth of the crystalline lens, which tends to push the entire iris diaphragm forward when the endocorneal angle of the anterior chamber is less than 20 degrees in width. Then a state of narrow-angle glaucoma is said to exist (Fig. 5-2). Often the trigger mechanism that brings about closure of a critically narrowed angle is dilation of the pupil. Dilation of the pupil relaxes the iris and causes tissue to bunch up toward the base of the iris, thereby effectively blocking off the angle structures. The iris may become adherent to the lens and may bow forward, the so-called iris bombé (Fig. 5-3). In this situation, the pupil is blocked so that the aqueous pressure from the posterior chamber bows the iris forward and blocks the angle of the anterior chamber, preventing the outflow of fluid. Abrupt onset is characteristic: An attack of acute angle-closure glaucoma can become fully developed within 30 to 60 minutes. Commonly, the attack begins under conditions leading to pupillary dilation, for example, fear, emotional arousal, or conditions of dark adaptation (as in movie theaters). Many an attack may be precipitated by dilation during an eye examination. The pain can vary from feeling discomfort and fullness around the eyes to a severe, prostrating pain that can radiate to the back of the head and down toward the teeth, often with nausea and vomiting. Vision is reduced to mere light perception. The cornea may appear steamy and hazy because of tiny water droplets in the superficial layers of the cornea. The iris may appear dull, gray, and patternless because of the edema. The pupil is typically dilated and may be oval and usually does not respond to light. Tension will be extremely high, in the range of 50 to 60 mm Hg or higher. The halos that often

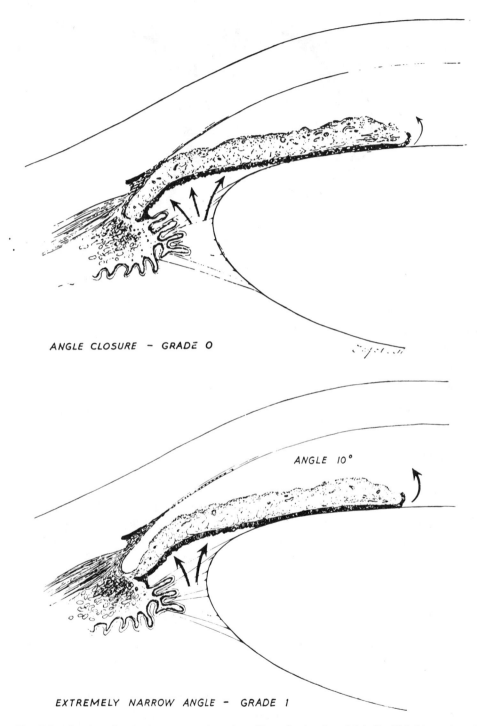

ANGLE CLOSURE — GRADE 0

ANGLE 10°

EXTREMELY NARROW ANGLE — GRADE 1

Fig. 5-2   Grading of angles by name and number. (From Becker B and Schaffer RN: Diagnosis and therapy of the glaucomas, ed 2, St Louis, 1965, The CV Mosby Co.)

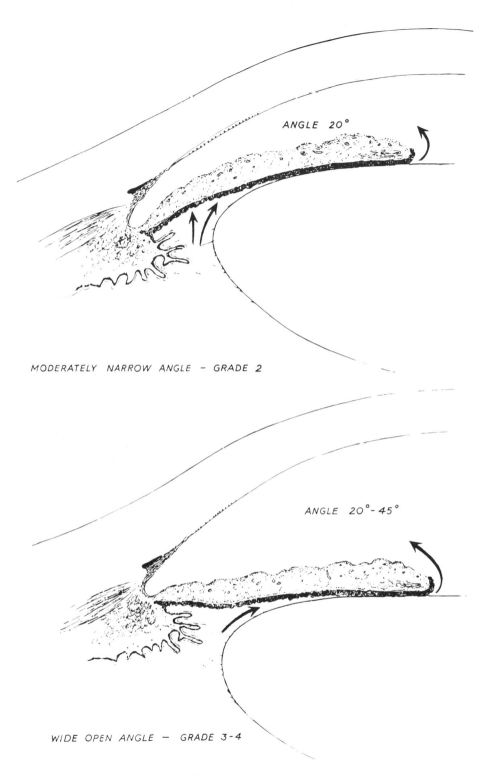

ANGLE 20°

MODERATELY NARROW ANGLE — GRADE 2

ANGLE 20°- 45°

WIDE OPEN ANGLE — GRADE 3-4

Fig. 5-2, cont'd Grading of angles by name and number.

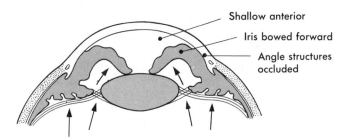

Fig. 5-3   Pupillary block glaucoma. The pressure in the posterior chamber exceeds that of the anterior chamber. The iris is bowed forward (iris bombé) and occludes the angle structures. Without treatment the iris becomes permanently adherent to the angle structures, and intractable secondary glaucoma ensues.

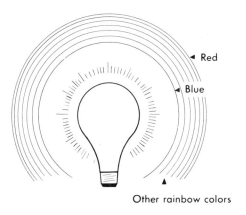

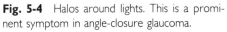

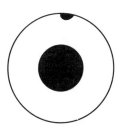

Fig. 5-4   Halos around lights. This is a prominent symptom in angle-closure glaucoma.

Fig. 5-5   Peripheral iridectomy. A small wedge of iris is removed from its base.

appear around lights are caused by the edema of the cornea and may occur before the severe pain that ensues (Fig. 5-4). They are typically composed of two colored rings, an inner blue-violet ring and an outer yellow-red ring.

   Treatment. The treatment of angle-closure glaucoma is surgical. A laser iridectomy or surgical iridectomy may be performed to relieve pupillary block and allow the anterior chamber to deepen (Fig. 5-5). If the attack is not prolonged and extensive adhesions have not been formed between the iris and angle structure, this procedure is usually curative. The argon and Nd-YAG laser, however, have virtually eliminated the need and risk of surgical procedures. When one eye has been subject to an attack of angle-closure glaucoma, the other eye has a strong chance of experiencing a similar attack. For this reason, most surgeons prefer to do a prophylactic iridotomy by laser on the healthy eye to avoid the hazards of acute angle-closure glaucoma.

Medical therapy for angle-closure glaucoma is useful only as a prelude to surgery or laser treatment. Its object is to lower intraocular pressure and open the blocked angle so that subsequent surgery can be performed more safely and with greater ease. Carbonic anhydrase inhibitors such as acetazolamide (Diamox) or methazolamide (Neptazene) are used to temporarily lower the intraocular pressure. Beta blockers such as Timolol, Betagen, or Betoptic work in conjunction with carbonic anhydrase inhibitors to lower intraocular pressure by stopping the inflow. Miotic agents are used to pull the iris away from the peripheral angle. Pilocarpine 2% or carbachol 1.5% or 3% is instilled in the affected eye several times, 5 minutes apart. In addition to carbonic anhydrase inhibitors, various hypertonic agents have been used to gain a more prompt and rapid reduction of intraocular pressure. The agents most commonly used today are (1) mannitol, given in a dose of 1 to 2 g/kg of body weight intravenously, and (2) glycerin, given in a dose of 1.5 g/kg of body weight orally with orange juice. Pain killers may be utilized. Treatment should begin as soon as the diagnosis is made.

Primary open-angle glaucoma

Primary open-angle glaucoma is a relentless bilateral chronic disease. In most cases, glaucoma develops in middle life or later and the onset is gradual and asymptomatic. The cause of the disorder is obstruction of the outflow of aqueous humor in the trabecular meshwork. Most cases of primary open-angle glaucoma are caused by an inability of aqueous fluid to leave the eye and not by an overproduction of aqueous fluid (Fig. 5-6). No symptoms occur until the disease has progressed or until an excavated disc or elevated tension is detected on routine eye examination. Diagnosis of this condition depends on three objective signs: (1) increased intraocular pressure, (2) cupping of the disc (Figs. 5-7 and 5-8), and (3) field defects (Figs. 5-9 through 5-14). The optic disc often will reveal the diagnosis of raised intraocular pressure. The cumulative effect of

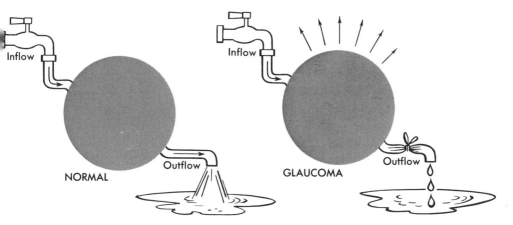

Fig. 5-6 Obstruction of aqueous outflow causes an elevation of intraocular tension.

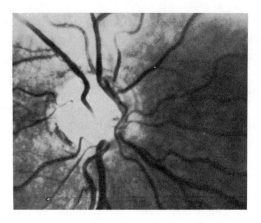

Fig. 5-7 Cupping of the optic disc. Note the dip of the vessels as they traverse the temporal margin of the disc.

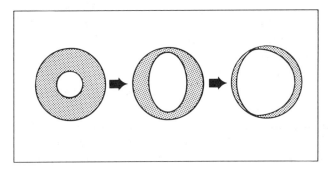

Fig. 5-8 Progressive cupping or increasing cup-to-disc ratio in the right eye in glaucoma

sustained pressure results in atrophy of the optic nerve at its entrance into the eye. These changes consist of pallor and cupping of the optic disc. Cupping usually manifests itself on the temporal aspect of the optic disc, resulting in the retinal vessels dipping down over a saucerized edge at the margin of the disc, instead of running across it smoothly. The disc also appears pale. The optic disc should be evaluated as follows:

1 *Cup/disc ratio.* Most patients have a cup/disc ratio (C/D ratio) of less than 0.5. A higher C/D ratio or asymmetry between the discs is suggestive of glaucoma.

2 *Color of the neural rim.* A normal neural rim will have a pink color and should be similar in both eyes. In advanced glaucoma the neural rim is pale with compression of the fine capillaries (see Fig. 5-7).

The patient should be followed with visual field assessments. Here it is necessary to use a tangent screen or Goldman perimeter to detect early field changes. The patient's

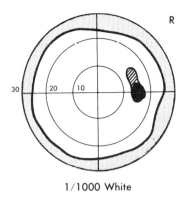

1/1000 White

Fig. 5-9 Enlargement of the normal blind spot.

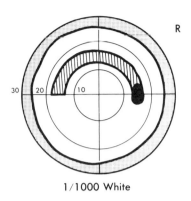

1/1000 White

Fig. 5-10 Nerve fiber bundle defect.

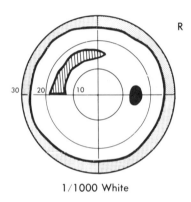

1/1000 White

Fig. 5-11 Arcuate defect, or Bjerrum's sco-toma, not attached to blind spot.

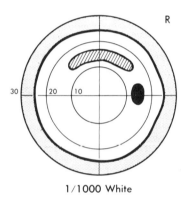

1/1000 White

Fig. 5-12 Arcuate defect, or Bjerrum's sco-toma, not attached to blind spot.

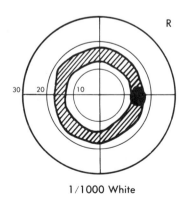

1/1000 White

Fig. 5-13 Double arcuate scotoma, producing a ring field defect.

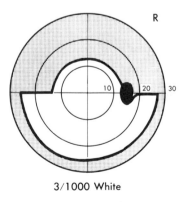

3/1000 White

Fig. 5-14 Advanced glaucomatous field defect.

central field remains relatively good until late in the disease, while the peripheral vision gradually erodes and becomes constricted to tunnel vision. The disease is painless and often symptomless and must be picked up by tonometry and retinal examination.

Secondary glaucoma

Secondary glaucoma occurs because of other diseases within the eye. Conditions that can lead to secondary glaucoma are:

- Dislocation of the crystalline lens
- Swollen crystalline lens
- Scar tissue or peripheral anterior synechiae (adhesions) between the iris and trabecular meshwork
- Posterior synechiae attachment to the crystalline lens; adhesions are brought about by chronic iritis; invasions by tumors of the iris, ciliary body, and choroid may result in secondary open-angle glaucoma
- Trauma with recession of the iris
- Neovascular glaucoma with a network of vessels that may occur with diabetes and central retinal vein occlusion
- Drug-induced glaucoma by such drugs as the corticosteroids
- Lens-induced glaucoma, by far advanced cataracts that have increased in size or in which denatured lens protein has leaked through an intact capsule, causing a response of macrophages that block the angle; dislocated lenses may occur from trauma, Marfan's syndrome, or hemocystinuria

Congenital glaucoma

Congenital glaucoma is rare. Often parents are unaware that their baby has anything wrong with the eye. The child appears extremely sensitive to light and tears profusely. Eventually, with prolonged pressure, corneal haziness may occur as a result of corneal edema. Because the coats of the eye are distensible in early infancy, the increased intraocular pressure causes progressive enlargement of the infantile eye and cornea. Most infantile corneas measure less than 10.5 mm in horizontal diameter. A measurement over 12 mm is considered diagnostic of congenital glaucoma. These eyes, hazy and enlarged, appear so grotesque that the term buphthalmos, or ox eye, has been commonly applied to designate this condition.

CATARACTS

The most common cause of painless, progressive loss of vision today is cataracts. They occur more commonly in the elderly but are by no means restricted to this group. The patient with a cataract sees as if he were looking through a frosted window. Objects may start to become hazy because of the irregular refraction of light through the changing crystalline lens of the eye. The patient perceives objects with an amber cast. Cataracts are usually bilateral, but their development may be asymmetrical, so the patient may have a moderate reduction of vision or none at all in one eye and a severe visual reduction in the other. It is only when the cataract becomes mature or totally opaque that the vision drops to the point of mere light perception and projection. Most patients who have access to a medical center may have their cataracts removed before they become mature. In areas were medical facilities are not available, cataracts are the leading cause of blindness. Until the cataracts have sufficiently advanced, there may develop increased myopia so that the individual may be able to see up close better than he sees in the distance. Cataracts may be of small size and faint in density so that the transmission of light is not appreciably affected. However, it may be large and opaque so that the light cannot gain entry into the interior of the eye. The procedure for surgical removal depends on whether the cataract interferes with the patient's ability to function or endangers the eye. In many cases, ambient lighting may affect the visual level. The patient may see well in a dimly lit room. Once the patient is affected by sunshine and glare and the pupil becomes small, a central opacity can cause a considerable amount of difficulties for many individuals. Contrast sensitivity is another method of determining defects in vision that cannot normally be recorded on the Snellen chart.

There are many ways of defining and classifying cataracts. They may be classified as to their *cause,* for example:

Galactosemia cataract

Steroid-induced cataract

Metabolic cataract

Radiation cataract

Glass-blower cataract

Traumatic cataract

Electric cataract

One may classify them as to their *time of onset:*

Embryonal cataract

Congenital cataract

Juvenile cataract

Late onset age-related cataract

or, by the *anatomic position* in the lens, such as:

Nuclear

Sutural

Zonular

Posterior subcapsular

or, according to their *stage of development:*

Immature cataract

Mature cataract

Hypermature cataract

Intumescent cataract

Age-related cataract

This is the most common type of cataract that occurs. With age, the lens fibers become more compact in the central nuclear portion of the lens and so a hard nuclear sclerotic crystalline lens occurs. As nuclear sclerosis advances, vision is affected and myopia may

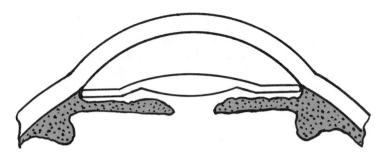

Fig. 5-15   Anterior chamber, angle-fixated intraocular lens.

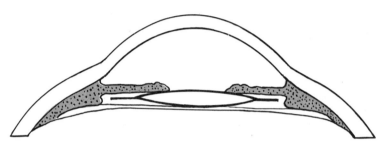

Fig. 5-16   Posterior chamber intraocular lens.

be induced. A shift to a yellow color of the lens occurs. In late stages, complications from an intumescent cataract may occur, such as glaucoma and lens-induced uveitis.

The method for surgical removal has changed dramatically in the past several years from the intracapsular operation performed a number of years ago. Surgeons today have switched over to extracapsular procedures and phacoemulsification. Both procedures leave the posterior capsule intact to prevent damage by unwanted ultraviolet light to the macula and to permit a safer place to insert a posterior chamber implant. Implant surgery is the exception, with only rare indications for a nonimplant procedure. Occasionally, if a patient has had surgery by the intracapsular method, an anterior chamber lens may be used or a posterior chamber lens may be required to be sewn into the sclera. Phacoemulsification, while still not performed by the majority of ophthalmologists at present, is becoming an increasingly popular procedure with a small incision and rapid recovery rate. Outpatient surgery is the current popular method for most cataract procedures unless there is some contraindication and the patient requires hospitalization because of health reasons (Figs. 5-15 and 5-16).

RETINAL DETACHMENT

Retinal detachments are usually tear induced (*rhegmatogenous*, from Greek *rhegma*, hole) (Fig. 5-17). The mechanisms for a detachment are the presence of a retinal hole

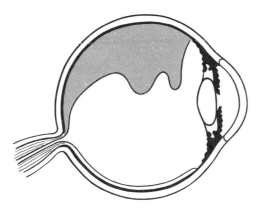

Fig. 5-17   Retinal detachment.

or tear and liquid vitreous that gets under the sensory layers of the retina and provides a fluid wedge under the retina. Some force to effect the separation may be produced by minor trauma or even eye movement. In the elderly, tears or holes may occur because of senile degeneration of the retina. If aphakia is present, the fluid and gel components of the vitreous are often disrupted by the original surgery, particularly if there was vitreous loss, and adds to the risk of a detachment. In myopia, characterized by an increase in axial length, there is a greater tendency for retinal and vitreous peripheral degenerative changes to occur and for a higher incidence of retinal detachments. When the retina detaches, it is not truly a detachment of the entire retina but a splitting of the retina as the pigment layer of the retina remains attached to the choroid, while the anterior nine out of ten layers detach from the posterior pigment layer. The vitreous wedges itself between the split layers. In the management of potential detachments, holes and tears are usually sealed if detected early by laser photocoagulation. The fellow eye may be also treated. Detecting a retinal tear may take place at the time of a routine examination. A common symptom is the shower of floating spots. Flashes of light or floaters may precede a rhegmatogenous retinal detachment. This may be caused by small, broken blood vessels that have liberated free red blood cells, which in turn casts a shadow on the retina. Vitreous traction is the major cause of retinal tears and almost always occurs spontaneously. At times, the retina can be detached and no holes found (nonrhegmatogenous). This could be the result of trauma or inflammation. The most sinister cause of a nonrhegmatogenous detachment is a malignant melanoma.

Symptoms may also be absent in the case of detachment until a retinal veil occurs, in which a shadow appears on one or other side of the eye. Some patients complain of light flashes; others may complain of a veil or curtain that ascends or descends before one's vision. Some individuals lose their vision if the macula is involved. This requires immediate repair. Most procedures today are successful if the condition is detected early.

Examination with the ophthalmoscope in the case of a retinal detachment reveals a rippling gray retina that is thrown into folds in one or the other quadrant. This membrane is translucent and obscures the details of the pigment, epithelium and choroid and often trembles with each movement of the eye. Careful search will often reveal a small hole. Each eye must be examined, since the other eye often has some retinal holes or adhesions that may be dealt with by laser.

Defects of the retina may be considered a break if there is a full-thickness retinal defect, a hole if there is a round, atrophic break, tear if the break is caused by vitreous retraction pulling on the retina, or a flap or horseshoe tear in which a strip of the retina is pulled by the vitreous. The retina may also degenerate at the periphery.

OCULAR MANIFESTATIONS OF THYROID DISORDERS

Ocular disease can be seen in patients with hyperthyroidism (excessive thyroid activity), hypothyroidism (depressed thyroid activity), and even euthyroidism (normal thyroid function after successful treatment for hyperthyroidism).

Hyperthyroid people tend to have a rapid pulse, shortness of breath, and a loss of weight. Hypothyroid people show a deceleration of activity and may be dull mentally, with a low voice, reduced pulse rate, dry skin, and a gain in weight.

Patients with a thyroid disorder and specific eye findings have a condition called Graves' disease. The etiologic factors of this condition are thought to be immunologic. A variety of tests can be employed for diagnosis of the thyroid condition: serum thyroxine, T_3 resin uptake, thyroid autoantibodies, thyrotropin-releasing hormone (TRH), and T_3 assay.

The ocular manifestations of Graves' disease include the following:

- *Lid lag.* This is one of the earliest findings. When the patient looks down, the lid tends to lag behind the downward moving eye.
- *Lid retraction.* The lids may leave a clear white space between the lid margins, both upper and lower, and the limbus.
- *Exophthalmos, or protrusion of the eye.* Using either the Hertel or Krahn exophthalmometer, the degree of protrusion can be measured. It is usually between 20 and 28 mm of exophthalmos. The forward displacement of the globe is caused by an increase in the bulk of ocular muscles and orbital fat swelling. A computed tomography scan will document the swollen extraocular muscles.
- *Exposure keratitis.* Lid retraction and proptosis lead to exposure of the cornea and its consequent drying effect.
- *Motility disturbance.* Limitation of eye movements can ensue because of direct involvement of the extraocular muscles. The cellular infiltration of these muscles can lead to fibrosis, with a resultant tethering effect on their function. The most common muscles affected, in descending order of frequency, are the inferior rectus, medial rectus, superior rectus, and lateral rectus.
- *Disc edema.* Flow through the optic nerve can be slowed by orbital compression. This can lead to disc edema. The swollen nerve is commonly a prelude to optic atrophy with a permanent visual loss.

Management of Graves' disease involves both the internist, to treat and manage the thyroid condition, and the ophthalmologist, to deal with the ocular complications. Guanethidine eyedrops, 10%, are often helpful in reducing the lid retraction, which is cosmetically disfiguring. The lid retraction can also be aided surgically by cutting Müller's muscle and a section of the levator palpebrae superioris.

Exposure keratitis can be managed by liberal lubrication with artificial tears and ointment. Therapy is indicated if the orbital congestion causes a decrease in either color vision or central vision, or a defect on visual field testing. Therapy may consist of systemic steroids, orbital radiation, or an orbital decompression (removing a wall of the orbit) to reduce the severe orbital pressure. If double vision results, muscle surgery can be used to relax the muscles and align the eyes.

STRABISMUS

Strabismus is a failure of the eyes to spontaneously direct the gaze at the same object because of muscular imbalance. Orthoptics is the science that investigates the motor and sensory adaptations of strabismus and deals with nonsurgical treatment to help patients regain the ability to use both eyes together normally to obtain comfortable, binocular single vision. In evaluating strabismus, one should note (1) age of onset and the type of onset (rapid or slow), (2) whether the turn is intermittent or constant, (3) whether one eye turns at all times, or whether either eye alternately turns, (4) if strabismus is more apparent with close work or when looking in the distance, (5) precipitating causes before onset of squint such as illness or trauma, (6) family history of strabismus, (7) any previous therapy for treatment of strabismus, (8) birth trauma, and (9) general health and past health.

The Hirschberg test is a gross method for determining the presence or absence of the strabismus and its magnitude. The examiner shines a light at the patient's eyes and notes the position of the reflex of light, which normally falls on a slightly nasal spot off the center of the pupil of each eye. If this reflex is temporally placed in one eye and is normal in the other eye, the child obviously has an esotropia or convergent strabismus (Fig. 5-18). Each millimeter of deviation from the normal position of the light reflex represents approximately 7 degrees to be displaced. If the light falls on the nasal side of one pupil and on the center of the fellow pupil, then the eye is said to diverge and there is present an exotropia, or divergent strabismus. A more sophisticated way of measuring the deviation is to use prisms and alternately cover one eye or the other eye. The strength of the prism will represent the deviation of the eye when no further movement occurs on alternate cover. The Worth four-dot test is used to detect the presence of fusion or suppression in one eye (see Skills, Chapter 3).

AMBLYOPIA

Amblyopia exists when there is a difference of two or more lines in the visual acuity of the eyes. The incidence of amblyopia is approximately 2.5% of the population in which the vision is reduced in the affected eye to 20/40 or less. Amblyopia is a loss of vision in which no organic pathologic condition is seen in the eye or its extensions in the brain.

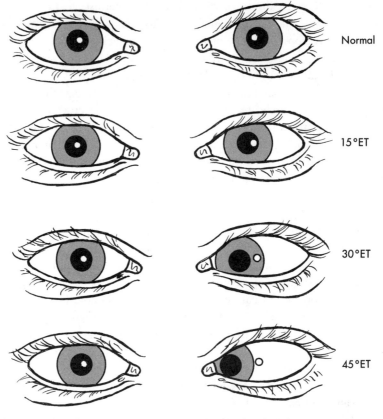

Normal

15°ET

30°ET

45°ET

Fig. 5-18   Hirschberg's method of estimating deviation.

It is most common in strabismus and is the result of longstanding suppression of the turned eye to avoid diplopia. It also may occur when a large refractive error exists in one eye and has been undetected in childhood. It also may occur in congenital cataracts and traumatic cataracts in early infancy, and vision is blocked. If the amblyopia is profound and longstanding, eccentric fixation may result. In eccentric fixation, a new focussing point is selected other than the fovea and takes over the function of the macula. Because the new point is off-center or eccentric to the fovea, visual acuity is extremely poor because of the low density of cones.

Amblyopic treatment is based on occlusion of the good eye to permit the amblyopic or lazy eye to see full time. Occlusion is maintained during all waking hours until the visual acuity is equal. Children between the ages of 4 and 7 usually require a much longer period of therapy to produce improvement in visual acuity than do younger children. After this age, usually occlusion does not produce any results. In any event, if 3 months of constant occlusion does not produce sufficient improvement in vision, usually occlusion therapy is discontinued.

Diagnosing common eye disorders

Many eye disorders are visible on external examination. The careful observer will visually distinguish many of the fine points involved in the diagnosis of these disorders by the naked eye or with low-power magnification. The purpose of this section is to make diagnosticians of students and to enrich the study of common eye disorders.

THE CONJUNCTIVA
Hyperemia

Hyperemia, or redness, of the conjunctiva is perhaps the most common condition seen. The offensive redness is merely caused by dilation of the normal vascular channels in the conjunctiva. It can be caused by such transitory and innocuous events as exposure to dust, wind, or air pollutants, fatigue, excessive reading, exposure to strong light or heat, poor ventilation, excessive dryness, and even the moderate consumption of alcoholic beverages. Many people equate red eyes with infection or inflammation and become alarmed. It is for this reason that proprietary medications to "get the red out" are so successful with their media advertising. Many people think that by getting the red out they are nipping a disease process in the bud, as well as removing a socially unacceptable red eye.

Transitory redness of the eyes requires no treatment because it is not a disease. People who find some relief with the use of eyewashes or astringent drops get only a temporary abatement of their symptoms and become addicted to drops for the rest of their lives. When the medication wears off, the conjunctival vessels have a tendency to dilate again, so that the redness becomes even more prominent than before.

Subconjunctival hemorrhage

Subconjunctival hemorrhage is caused by a ruptured conjunctival blood vessel. It usually causes an irregular red patch because of pooling of blood under the conjunctiva. Its

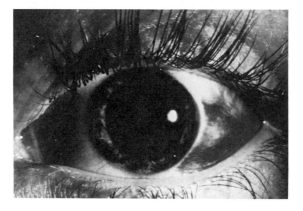

Fig. 5-19   Subconjunctival hemorrhage.

appearance is particularly gruesome and alarming because it is accentuated by the white of the sclera (Fig. 5-19). Invariably, collection of blood, like any other bruise under the skin, spreads and seems to enlarge as the blood is disseminated. Eventually the blood pigment breaks down to its component parts until it is absorbed. This process can take anywhere from 7 days to 3 weeks, depending on the size of the hemorrhage.

Subconjunctival hemorrhage occurs most often in elderly patients who are diabetic or who have hypertension, but commonly no cause can be found. A predisposing cause appears to be events that cause a sudden rise in venous pressure, such as coughing, straining, lifting, sneezing, or vomiting. There is no treatment for this condition, which is entirely innocuous, other than reassurance. Occasionally a subconjunctival hemorrhage is part of a general bleeding disorder, but it must be emphasized that such an event is rare.

Conjunctivitis (see Fig. 9-9)

Conjunctivitis is an inflammation of the conjunctiva characterized by redness of the conjunctiva, swelling, a discharge that can be watery or purulent, and congestion of the tissues (Fig. 5-20). The patient commonly complains of a burning or grittiness of the eyes. Characteristically, the discharge accumulates during sleep, and its resultant drying on the lashes makes the lids difficult to open in the morning. Usually the lids have to be bathed to open the eyes.

Conjunctivitis may have an infectious, allergic, or toxic cause. The most common infectious agents are viruses, bacteria, and chlamydial organisms. A virus is the most common cause of conjunctivitis. Unlike bacterial or chlamydial conjunctivitis, the discharge is characteristically watery. Adenovirus is the most common viral conjunctivitis. Certain serotypes of this infectious agent may be responsible for causing epidemic keratoconjunctivitis (EKC) or pharyngoconjunctival fever (PCF). EKC is highly contagious

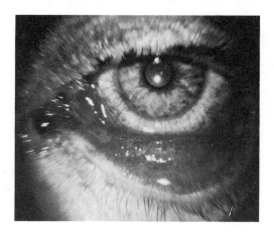

Fig. 5-20 Conjunctivitis.

and is often associated with epidemic outbreaks in a localized area. This disease is characterized by conjunctival and corneal involvement. PCF differs from EKC in that patients will usually exhibit symptoms of a sore throat, just preceding or at the same time as their ocular symptoms.

Staphylococcus aureus is the most common cause of bacterial conjunctivitis. The organism is also responsible for such common conditions as boils or impetigo of the skin. Gonococcal conjunctivitis can be a severe infection resulting in blindness if appropriate treatment is delayed. The disease can be seen in newborns who contact the organism while traveling through the birth canal. The sequelae of neonatal conjunctivitis can be so devastating that it is mandatory in most countries for either antibacterial drops or 1% silver nitrate to be placed into the lower conjunctival sac of all newborns immediately after birth. Gonococcal conjunctivitis can also be seen in adults and is characterized by a significant purulent discharge. These patients and their sexual contacts need to be evaluated for a venereal disease that was probably the source for the conjunctivitis. *Haemophilus influenzae,* another bacterial organism, can cause pinkeye, especially in children.

Chlamydial conjunctivitis can be caused by inclusion conjunctivitis of trachoma. The disease is characterized by a red eye and often a mucoid discharge. Inclusion conjunctivitis is the more prevalent of the two in North America and is seen in newborns and young adults. Trachoma is a more severe disease that can give rise to extensive scarring of the lids, conjunctiva, and cornea. It is epidemic in some parts of the world, such as North Africa, the Middle East, and South Asia, where poor hygiene, poor sanitation, deficient diets, and crowding are the norm. It is a major cause of blindness in the world.

The features that distinguish acute conjunctivitis, acute iritis, and acute glaucoma are shown in Fig. 5-21 and Table 5-1. Smears and cultures may be required in selected cases, especially in patients with ophthalmia neonatorum (conjunctivitis of the newborn), membranous conjunctivitis (diphtheria), and purulent conjunctivitis (gonococcal).

Table 5-1   Differential diagnosis

	Acute conjunctivitis	Acute iritis	Acute glaucoma
Pain	None to grittiness or foreign body sensation	Moderate to severe	Severe and radiating
Discharge	Watery or purulent	None	Tearing only
Sensitivity to light (photophobia)	Mild	Severe	Moderate
Cornea	Bright and clear	Clear or hazy	Hazy
Pupil	Normal	Constricted or small	Dilated, oval, fixed to light
Intraocular pressure	Normal	Usually normal	Elevated

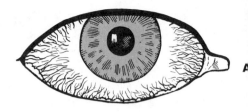

Acute conjunctivitis

Fig. 5-21 **A,** Acute conjunctivitis, with discharge, injection greater in the fornix, clear cornea, and pupil normal in size. **B,** Acute glaucoma, with tearing, extreme injection of entire eye, hazy cornea, and pupil that is dilated, oval, and fixed to light. **C,** Iritis, with no discharge, circumcorneal injection, clear to slightly hazy cornea, and small pupil.

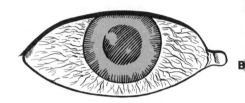

Acute glaucoma

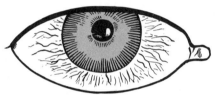

Iritis

Allergic conjunctivitis is basically a hypersensitivity reaction. It may occur as a component of hay fever or as an independent ocular allergy. There may be large formations of papules or cobblestones under the eyelid (Fig. 5-22). At times the conjunctivitis may be an allergic response to an invading organism, such as the tuberculosis, protein, or staphylococcal bacillus. Contact allergies to drugs are a common occurrence and one of the main reasons why an inflammation can progress despite the copious applications of medication. Neomycin and sulfur preparations are particularly sensitizing.

Chemical conjunctivitis is often seen in the summer and is caused by irritation from chlorine in swimming pools. It may also be seen in industrial workers after exposure to irritating fumes.

Obviously, the treatment of conjunctivitis depends on identifying its cause and applying the appropriate therapy. Local antibiotic drops that are effective for a bacterial conjunctivitis would obviously be of no value for a viral infection.

The diagnosis of conjunctivitis is largely made on clinical grounds and, if serious enough, enhanced with laboratory studies. For example, in a membranous conjunctivitis caused by diphtheria, swabs are taken from the discharge for a smear preparation, and samples are also cultured for growth identification and drug sensitivity. Routine cultures and sensitivity tests are rarely done because the time lag in obtaining the re-

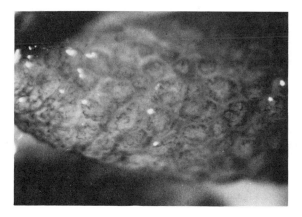

Fig. 5-22 Vernal conjunctivitis—cobblestone formation of upper tarsus, noted when lid is everted.

sults of such investigation does not warrant the delay in treatment. Where there is serious potential in conjunctivitis, the ophthalmologist will do appropriate laboratory investigations but will institute therapy first. If the trial of therapy does not work, it can later be altered when the precise etiologic agent has been identified and the exact drug to which it is sensitive has been determined.

Pinguecula/pterygium

A *pinguecula* is a triangular, wedge-shaped thickening of the conjunctiva, usually found encroaching on the nasal limbus. If it invades the cornea, it is then called a *pterygium* (Fig. 5-23). These lesions appear as yellowish or white vascularized masses. They are common in tropical climates where people spend a great deal of time outdoors, where they are exposed to sunlight and the harmful effects of ultraviolet light. Pinguecula do not usually cause symptoms. Occasionally they may cause some irritation or may be a cosmetic blemish. Treatment with artificial tears, vasoconstrictors, or rarely, surgical

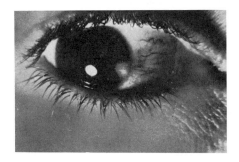

Fig. 5-23 Pterygium actively invading the cornea.

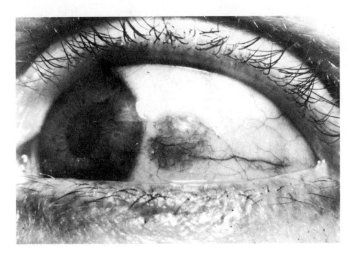

Fig. 5-24 Pigmented nevus of the conjunctiva. (From Liebman SD and Gellis SS, editors: The pediatrician's ophthalmology, St Louis, 1966, The CV Mosby Co.)

excision may be indicated. Pterygia can occasionally extend across the cornea and eventually encroach on the visual axis and cause loss of vision. If there is documented evidence of growth, or if the lesion is close to the visual axis, then surgical excision is indicated. Unfortunately, there is a high incidence of recurrence, so surgical removal is commonly combined with beta-radiation to minimize recurrences.

Conjunctival nevus

A nevus is a benign neoplasm that appears on the conjunctiva at birth or in early childhood. The most common appearance is that of a flat, slightly elevated brown spot (Fig. 5-24). It usually becomes pigmented late in childhood or in adolescence. It is uncommon for a nevus to become malignant. This condition should be differentiated from the acquired pigmented lesion that can occur by the age of 40 to 50 and that can, with growth, turn into a malignant melanoma.

THE CORNEA

The cornea, which forms the anterior sixth of the globe and functionally is the main refracting surface of the eye, is the most vulnerable structure to injury or inflammation. It is almost completely exposed so that it receives the brunt of chemical injuries to the eye, foreign bodies, particulate matter, and organisms that can invade it from such contiguous sources as the conjunctiva and the lacrimal sac. It is avascular tissue, which means that it is robbed of the defense mechanisms that normally are marshalled against any inflammatory insult elsewhere in the body. The corneal epithelium provides a strong barrier against bacterial invasion. The integrity of this surface is best appreciated by applying fluorescein to its surface and noting any defects in the integrity of this layer by the accumulation of fluorescein pools.

Keratoconus

Keratoconus is a developmental abnormality in which the cornea progressively becomes thinned centrally and bulges forward in a conical fashion. It is usually bilateral and occurs more often in females than in males. It creates irregular corneal astigmatism that defies correction by ordinary spectacles.

The diagnosis may be made by slit lamp examination, by the keratometer or retinoscope, which shows the presence of irregular corneal astigmatism, or by use of a keratoscope or Placido's disk, which reflects the images of disordered and irregular concentric circles on the surface of the cornea. Rigid contact lenses have been used to correct the visual defect. If the patient is unable to be fitted properly with contact lenses because of high irregular astigmatism, keratoplasty is necessary to restore vision.

Herpes simplex keratitis

Herpes simplex keratitis is a common corneal inflammatory disorder created by the herpes simplex virus, which is the offending agent of the common cold sore. The symptoms are relatively mild and consist of an irritating foreign body sensation, mild tearing with no frank pus or purulent discharge, and some haziness of vision accompanied by sensitivity to light. The classic herpes lesion is the dendritic figure, which, when stained with fluorescein, reveals a branchlike erosion of the cornea, sometimes as a single lesion or as multiple disturbances (Fig. 5-25).

The virus will remain dormant in the sensory nerves to the face, where it can be aroused by a variety of precipitating factors. These factors include the presence of emotional stress, trauma, menstruation, sunlight, or the use of steroid drugs either locally or systemically. The virus, when aroused, will travel down the sensory nerves to the face, lids, conjunctiva, and cornea to produce a recurrence of the disease. These recurrences

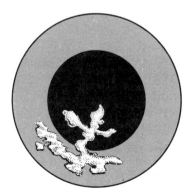

Fig. 5-25 Dendritic figure typical of herpes simplex keratitis.

may be common, adding insult to each previous episode, so that reduction of vision over the years is a common complication. If only the epithelium were involved, no scarring would occur. However, the inflammatory process commonly extends deep down toward the stroma, which heals with vascular proliferation from the limbus and results in corneal scarring.

This condition is dangerous diagnostically because it appears to be a simple conjunctivitis. Many patients treat themselves or are treated by their family physicians with antibiotics for a period of several days before the patient arrives in the ophthalmologist's office. Local antibiotics are of no value in this condition because it is caused by a virus. In many instances, self-medication severely aggravates the condition, since many antibiotic preparations are coupled with steroids, which cause the virus to proliferate even more, thus ensuring the spread of the ulcer and further necrosis of tissue.

The treatment of herpes keratitis is instillation of trifluridine (Viroptic) drops, or IDU or vidarabine (Vira-A) ointment. The cornea usually heals in 7 to 14 days in approximately 85% of cases. Some practitioners prefer to remove the offending virus by scraping off the diseased epithelium. This can be done at the slit lamp with a dull blade.

Superficial punctate keratitis

Superficial punctate keratitis consists of fine erosions in the corneal epithelium that can be appreciated with the slit lamp and fluorescein staining. These lesions are common and can be seen in dry-eye conditions, infections such as adenovirus and herpes simplex, and chemical injuries. Treatment varies, depending on the cause of the superficial punctate keratitis.

Herpes zoster ophthalmicus

Herpes zoster ophthalmicus is caused by a virus similar to the one that causes chickenpox in children. In the adult it is ushered in by a severe neuralgia-type pain, which usually includes the upper lid and extends upward beyond the brow to envelop the forehead through the scalp almost to the vertex of the head. Following the pain there is usually a vesicular eruption of the skin so that the skin surface becomes swollen, red, and heavily blistered (Fig. 5-26). The severe pain and vesicular phase last approximately 2 weeks. With healing, the skin is often pockmarked with deep, pitted scars, and sensitivity to normal sensation is depressed.

If the tip of the nose is involved with vesicles, it usually means that the nasocilliary nerve has been affected and that the underlying eye will also be affected by the herpes zoster virus. This occurs in about 50% of patients. Ocular disturbances include superficial and deep corneal ulcers, iritis, secondary glaucoma, and even paralysis of an extraocular muscle in the minority of instances.

Treatment may include the use of systemic steroids to decrease the scarring and pain that is so common after the inflammation has subsided. Ocular treatment may include topical steroids to decrease the inflammation and a cycloplegic agent to make the

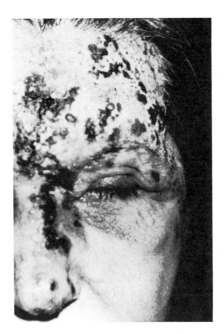

Fig. 5-26   Herpes zoster ophthalmicus.

patient more comfortable. Acyclovir is a new antiviral agent, administered in an oral form, that has been shown to be effective in shortening the course of disease in herpes zoster.

Marginal corneal ulcers

Marginal corneal ulcers are usually secondary to inflammation caused by the toxin of *Staphylococcus aureus* combined with cells and other mediators involved in the body's immunologic response. It is an extremely painful condition, and most patients believe that they have a large foreign body in their eye. There is marked redness around the eye, and there is usually a white infiltrate that extends from the limbus into the substance of the cornea for 2 to 4 mm. At times the cornea is ulcerated over the surface, but the epithelium may also be intact. The discharge is scant and usually watery.

Since this condition has an immunologic basis, it responds well to antibiotic-steroid medication. Other less common causes of marginal ulcers include nonimmunologic bacterial infections, herpes simplex, and inflammation secondary to a variety of systemic diseases, such as rheumatoid arthritis.

Recurrent corneal erosion

The typical history of recurrent corneal erosion is that the cornea is abraded by a fingernail, a branch of a tree, the edge of a piece of paper or cardboard, or any other organic agent. The actual injury heals temporarily, but a few days, weeks, or even months later the person experiences a complete recurrence of signs and symptoms of the original injury but does not have any recollection of having reinjured the eye. Invariably the symptoms occur in the morning and are thought to be caused by opening the eyes or by the trauma of rubbing the eyes, which removes the area of freshly healed epithelium on the cornea. The disorder is disabling because of the recurrent pain and is somewhat baffling because the features of the disorder are not evident in between attacks. The symptoms may last anywhere from 30 minutes to several hours or several days.

The use of hypertonic saline drops during the day and ointment at night is helpful in dehydrating the corneal epithelium, which makes it less likely to slough off. If this is unsuccessful, a therapeutic soft contact lens can be tried. A new treatment modality is anterior stromal puncture, in which a fine needle is used to make multiple puncture marks in the outer third of the cornea. This technique decreases the recurrence rate by forming stronger bonds between the epithelium and the underlying tissue.

THE LIDS (see Figs. 9-29 through 9-34)

Certain anatomic features of the lids affect the manner of lid response. For instance, the skin of the lid, unlike that in the rest of the face, is extremely thin, loosely attached, and devoid of thick connective tissue and a fatty layer. Therefore any inflammatory swelling may cause the skin of the lid to balloon out and look puffy, while the weight of the collection of fluid is commonly sufficient to cause ptosis. The lid margins contain the openings of the meibomian glands (oil-secreting glands), as well as small sweat glands (glands of Moll). It is easy to understand why people who put eyeliner on their lid margins get recurrent cysts. They do so by obstructing the orifices of these tiny glands with cosmetic pigments. The cilia or eyelashes are strong, short, curved hairs arranged in two or more closely set rows. They are longer and more numerous on the upper lid than the lower. They have a protective effect, eliminating debris from the eye except when they are themselves caked by debris of a heavy application of mascara.

Chronic inflammation of the lid margins results in thickened, heavily vascularized lids. At times lashes will fall out and, even worse, grow aberrantly. Instead of curving

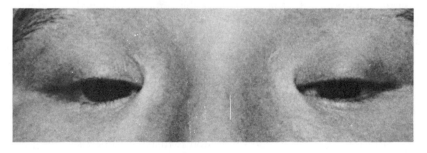

Fig. 5-27   Epicanthal folds.

out, they turn in to rub against the sensitive cornea, creating erosions and even ulcerations.

Normally, the upper lid just covers the upper millimeter or so of the cornea, whereas the lower lid skirts at its lower level. If the sclera is visible either above or below the cornea, it suggests either retraction of the lids or protrusion of the eye, which might be seen in hyperthyroidism, or caused by orbital inflammation or a tumor.

If the lid droops more than 1 to 2 mm over the cornea, the eye seems smaller by virtue of narrowing the palpebral fissure. This condition, called *ptosis*, is caused by the weakness of the muscles that elevate the upper lid (Müller's smooth muscle or the levator palpebrae superioris muscle). The condition may be congenital or acquired.

Epicanthus

Epicanthus is a common congenital variation in young Caucasian children. A vertical skin fold from the upper lid is present over the medial angle of the eye and the caruncle (Fig. 5-27). It makes the eyes seem closely set together, and many parents and general practitioners mistake this condition for strabismus. Invariably the condition is self-correcting with the growth of the base of the nose and the face. This variation persists throughout adult life with Oriental people. Surgical procedures eliminating this fold to make the eyes look rounder or more Caucasian are quite popular in Japan.

Entropion

An entropion is an in-turning of the lids; usually one of the lower lids is affected (Fig. 5-28). The spastic type is more common in elderly people than in youth. Its major disability is created by irritation to the cornea by the in-turned lashes. The inversion of the lid margin is a spasm of the orbicularis oculi, the washerlike muscle under the skin of the lid, and closes the eye. This muscle spasm is often induced by ocular inflammation or irritation. In an elderly person it is an easy feat for a spastic muscle to turn in on an atonic lid. A more severe form of entropion is caused by scarring, which can follow

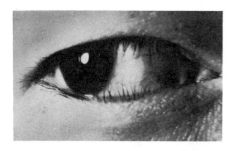

Fig. 5-28 Entropion with lashes invading the cornea.

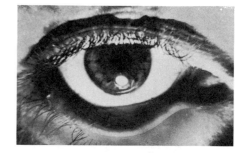

Fig. 5-29 Ectropion. The lower lid falls away from the globe so the punctum can no longer function as the exit portal for tears.

inflammation of the conjunctiva such as in ocular pemphigus, trachoma, lacerations of the lid, and chemical burns of the eye with attendant scarring. Again, surgery is required to remedy the condition.

The treatment of entropion is generally surgical, although temporary relief can be obtained by drawing the skin of the lower lid down toward the cheeks with adhesive tape. The surgery is safe, simple, and effective and is usually done with the patient under local anesthesia.

Ectropion

In this disorder the lid suffers a loss of tone and flops away from the eye so that the conjunctiva lining the inner surface of the lid becomes exposed, irritated, and thickened (Fig. 5-29). It occurs primarily in elderly people and is aggravated by attendant tearing as a result of aversion or stenosis of the punctum. The wiping away of tears from the lower lid makes the lower lid drop further, setting up a vicious cycle of tearing and progressive ectropion. Exposure of the conjunctiva causes burning and irritation and predisposes the eye to secondary inflammation. Again, the most common type is a result of senile atrophy of the lid structures, which causes the lids to stay outward. Scarring can also produce the same defect and is caused by the same conditions that create cicatricial entropion. An ectropion is a mechanical defect of the lids that can be remedied only by surgery.

Ptosis

In ptosis there is a conspicuous droop of the upper lid, and the opening of one eye seems smaller than the other (Fig. 5-30). Commonly the lid fold will be absent or smooth on the affected side. It is evident when the individual has to look up, because the lid on the affected side does not move upward with the globe as compared with the opposite normal side. If both lids are involved, a child will develop a characteristic head posture with the head thrown back and the upper lids elevated as a compensatory mechanism to raise the drooped eyelids. Treatment of the condition is invariably surgical. It is directed toward shortening the levator palpebrae superioris muscle, the primary elevator of the lid. Resection of a section of this muscle and advancement of its insertion strengthens it and increases its leverage.

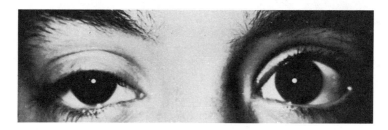

Fig. 5-30   Congenital ptosis, unilateral.

Exaggerated blink activity

This is a common condition seen especially in children. The sole feature is the presence of conspicuous repetitive blinking motions of the lids. Invariably the ocular examination reveals normal eyes. The rapid reflex blinking is thought to be the mechanism by which anxiety and restless motor activity are released in a young child. It clears by itself, and parents are best advised to ignore this self-limiting condition, which disappears more rapidly if it is ignored. Constant attention to these repetitive blinking motions only increases the child's anxiety.

A corollary to reflex blinking in the adult is tremor of the orbicularis oculi muscle. Many adults will complain of a fine lid flutter like a current going through the lower lid. Other than the annoying spontaneous twitch, it does not cause any other symptoms. The condition is usually caused by a mixture of tension and fatigue and disappears on its own. Rarely, it can be caused by serious conditions, such as Parkinson's disease, multiple sclerosis, and hyperthyroidism.

Blepharochalasis/dermatochalasis

Blepharochalasis is a condition that often drives middle-aged individuals to the plastic surgeon. It is caused by recurrent swelling of the upper lids and appears most prominently in the morning. The continuous stretching of the skin of the upper lids and the accumulation of edema cause the skin to lose its tone and hang lifelessly as a redundant fold or curtain over the upper lids. One disability is that it interferes with the application of eye makeup to the lids. In extreme cases it can even weigh on the lashes, creating a sensation of heaviness and ocular fatigue. It may cause restriction in the upper field of vision. At times this condition is accompanied by the protrusion of fat from behind the eye through the orbital septum just under the skin. These fat pads most prominently appear on the medial side of the upper lids and on the lower lids as rather large, unattractive mounds.

This condition is mainly, but not entirely, cosmetic and can be remedied surgically by removing the excess skin, removing the fat, and repairing the septum so that further protrusion of the retroorbital fat cannot occur.

Although blepharochalasis is largely innocuous, occasionally it is a manifestation of thyroid disease, kidney disorders, severe allergic reactions, or angioneurotic edema. This condition should be differentiated from dermatochalasis, which is predominantly an involutional aging change. Dermatochalasis is not a result of recurrent edema, but of loss of elastic tissue and relaxation of the fascial bands connecting the skin and underlying orbicularis muscle.

Trichiasis

In trichiasis, instead of being directed outward, the lashes turn in toward the eye, causing irritation and sometimes erosion and ulceration of the cornea. Trichiasis may be a result of scarring of the lid, which can be caused from previous injury, chemical burns to the lids, and severe lid inflammations. Simple epilation of the offending cilia is really a palliative measure, because the lashes tend to regrow aberrantly. If only a few lashes are irritating, their base can be cauterized by electrolysis. In more severe cases, a freezing technique applied to the base of the cilia, *cryosurgery*, or surgical reconstruction of the lid margin, may be necessary to remove the aberrant lashes that rub against the conjunctiva or cornea causing the irritation.

Blepharitis

Blepharitis is a common chronic inflammation of the lid margin. Patients usually complain of a sandy or itchy feeling of their eyes, especially in the morning. There is usually redness, as well as a thickening and irregularity of the lid margins. The disease may be seen at any age. The two most common types of chronic inflammation of the lids are staphylococcal blepharitis and seborrheic blepharitis. Seborrhea is a common cause of dandruff. Telltale diagnostic patches of seborrheic involvement in such patients are commonly seen in the medial aspect of the brows, the forehead, and sometimes behind the skin of the ear or on the nose. The base of the eyelash is usually caked with a greasy type of scale that comes off easily, leaving an intact lid margin.

At times the blepharitis can be infective in origin; when this is the case, it invariably is a result of the bacterium *Staphylococcus aureus*. The lid margins become ulcerated and congested, and adhesive exudate forms on the base of the follicles and on the lid margin. When the ulcerative scale is removed, it always reveals an ulcerative defect on the lid margin. The ulcerative type of blepharitis is more serious because if the inflammation reaches down to the base of the follicles, it can cause permanent scarring with either loss of lashes or misdirection of lash and regrowth with accompanying trichiasis. Also, the cosmetic consequences are undesirable because the lids become thickened, heavily vascularized, and unattractive.

External hordeolum (sty)/internal hordeolum

A sty is an acute suppurative inflammation of small sebaceous glands on the lid margin that empty their secretion into the hair follicles of the cilia. These glands are known as the glands of Zeis. An internal hordeolum is an acute inflammation of the sebaceous glands that reside in the tarsal plates—the meibomian glands. In the early stages of the inflammation, the affected gland becomes swollen, and the lid becomes red and edematous. An abscess forms with a small collection of pus, which usually points at the apex of one of these glands. Unless the suppuration is opened, the discomfort can be considerable. The inflammation is generally caused by invasion by *S. aureus*. It is a common affliction of young adults, but it can occur at all ages, especially in patients with blepharitis.

Treatment is primarily with hot compresses to rupture the gland in the early stage. If this is unsuccessful, one can incise and drain the hordeolum.

Chalazion

A chalazion is a chronic inflammatory granuloma of the large meibomian glands embedded in the tarsus of the lid. Chalazia may be multiple and can occur in the upper or

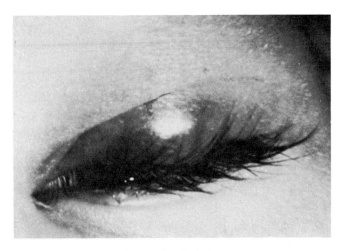

Fig. 5-31 Chalazion.

lower lids. Unlike the infectious cause of the internal and external hordeolum, chalazia are a result of a sterile process. Initially the orifice of the meibomian gland becomes occluded by a small inflammatory swelling, and the accumulative sebum ruptures the gland, creating a granulomatous type of inflammatory reaction in the lid itself. The lid becomes swollen, painful, and inflamed until eventually the inflammatory reaction is walled off and a cyst forms (Fig. 5-31). If the cyst is large and thickly walled, it may be opened surgically and evacuated with a curette and blunt dissection.

Sometimes in the early stages hot compresses will rupture it and can cause resolution of the inflammation. Many times the patient will come to the ophthalmologist after the inflammation has subsided with a nonpainful, localized swelling of the lid. The lesion may be surgically excised.

Tumors of the lid

Milia. Milia are small, white, slightly elevated cysts of the skin with a pedunuclated apex. They can create a cosmetic blemish when they appear in crops.

Xanthelasma. Yellowish fatty deposits, en plaque, occur in the upper and lower lids on the medial side. The condition is largely cosmetic, but it may indicate a more serious lipoid disorder, since it represents a deposit of circulating cholesterol or other lipids. The deposits can be destroyed or removed by trichloracetic acid, carbon dioxide snow, or surgery. The purpose of removing xanthelasma is strictly cosmetic.

Carcinoma. The most common malignant growth of the lid is the *basal cell carcinoma* (Fig. 5-32). It usually appears on the lower lid near the inner canthus, next on the lateral side of the lower lid, and finally and least commonly on the upper lids. The tumor typically has a raised ulcerated surface. Its margin is pearly white, and despite the appearance of tissue destruction, it rarely causes any symptoms. If the tumor is treated early with either radiotherapy or surgery, a complete cure can be effected. The tumor is invasive if it is not treated and tends to spread directly to the tissues surrounding it.

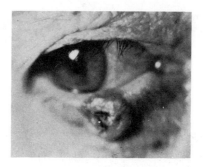

Fig. 5-32 Basal cell carcinoma of eyelid.

A much less common form of carcinoma is the squamous cell carcinoma. It has greater malignant potential and can spread to distant sites.

Seborrheic keratosis (senile verruca). This is one of the most common lesions involving the eyelid skin. It appears as a well-defined, small, elevated, brown to brownish black lesion on the eyelid, like a button flush on the skin surface. It is benign. It may be surgically removed for cosmetic reasons.

Keratoacanthoma. This is a benign lesion, but because of its rapid growth it is often mistaken for a malignancy. It grows rapidly but reaches maximum size in 6 to 8 weeks. There may be spontaneous regression, but it is usually excised.

Molluscum contagiosum. These are waxy, raised nodules, often with an umbilicated center. The lesions are caused by a member of the pox virus group. Toxic debris released from the lesion into the tears may give rise to a chronic conjunctivitis. The lesion usually has to be surgically excised.

LACRIMAL APPARATUS
Acute dacryoadenitis

Acute dacryoadenitis is an inflammation of the lacrimal gland that causes pain and discomfort in the upper outer portion of the orbit and swelling of the lid laterally. Eversion of the upper lid indicates a swollen, reddened gland on its lateral surface. Mumps and infectious mononucleosis are the usual systemic causes of this condition.

Lacrimal gland enlargement

Mass lesions of the lacrimal gland may manifest in a variety of ways. They may be painful or painless; they may be palpable, and they may be associated with swelling of the lid and ptosis. Enlargement of the lacrimal gland can be caused by tumor formation, such as the mixed tumor, adenoid cystic tumor, or lymphoma, or to a granulomatous inflammation.

Tearing

Tearing may be a result of *lacrimation*, which is excessive tear formation of the lacrimal gland, or they may be caused by epiphora, which is defective drainage of tears. Lacrimation may be a result of psychologic stimuli as an expression of grief or depression, or as a result of irritation of the eye from either wind or dust, or a result of irritative inflammatory disorders of the conjunctiva, cornea, or lids. These causes of lacrimation are usually self-evident and desist once the stimulus has stopped.

Persistent tearing, with overflow onto the cheek, is usually caused by obstruction somewhere in the lacrimal draining system from the punctum situated on the medial aspect of the lower lid through to the nasolacrimal duct. The patency of tear elimination can be tested in several ways. Fluorescein solution, 2%, instilled in the conjunctival sac normally disappears within 1 minute. A cotton swab placed in the nasal passages can usually prove the patency of the system as it becomes stained with fluorescein. Irrigation of the lacrimal system with saline solution is less physiologic but at least can demonstrate that tears will flow from the punctum to the nasolacrimal duct and empty into the nasal passages. If there is obstruction of the nasolacrimal canal, the tears forced through the lower canaliculus will reflux out through the upper punctum. This reflux of tears through the upper punctum is plainly visible. An additional point is that the person being tested will not taste the saline solution, which should be coming through the nose. Another test of tear function employs the use of saccharin solutions that are placed in the conjunctival sac. If tears are being eliminated, 1 or 2 minutes later the patency is proved by the patient indicating the taste of something in his throat.

It is also important to note the presence of apposition of the lower lid against the globe. Tearing can occur if the lower lid is not in contact with the globe as can be seen with medial ectropions.

Regardless of the cause, the treatment of tearing caused by defective drainage is largely surgical. The decision to operate depends on the distress of the patient created by the mechanical reflux of tears and the association of recurrent secondary infections.

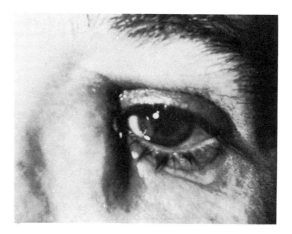

Fig. 5-33 Dacryocystitis. Note the marked swelling over the lacrimal sac.

Dacryocystitis

Dacryocystitis is an inflammation of the lacrimal sac and is indicated by an inflammatory swelling at the site of the sac. This inflamed swelling is seen as a visible red lump just below the caruncle overriding the inframedial aspect of the orbital bone (Fig. 5-33). Sometimes pressure over the sac will cause pus or mucoid material to regurgitate through the punctum. This condition usually results from the effects of stricture of a nasolacrimal duct arising from chronic inflammation, usually of nasal origin. Obstruction to the lower end of this duct can be caused by the presence of a nasal polyp and extreme deviation of the septum or a marked congestion of the inferior turbinate. Surgery, called *dacryocystorhinostomy* (DCR), is required to establish a new canal for the tears to flow to prevent stagnation.

Dry eyes

Tear formation is generally measured by the Schirmer test, in which a 35 mm by 5 mm strip of #41 Whatman filter paper or standardized paper is folded over the midportion of the lower lid. Generally, if 10 mm or more of the paper from the point of the fold becomes wet in a 5-minute period, tear formation is considered normal. This test measures both reflex and basic secretion.

The basic secretion test is done similarly, but only after a local anesthetic has been placed into the eye. This eliminates the reflex production of tears from the test and measures basal secretion.

A dry eye, referred to as *keratoconjunctivitis sicca,* is one deficient of tears, and is a far more serious problem than an eye bothered by an excess of tears. A deficiency of lacrimal secretion gives rise to chronic conjunctival irritation, which may be associated with erosions of the cornea and eventually corneal scarring.

If keratoconjunctivitis sicca is part of a general systemic disorder, which includes a variety of joint and skin diseases, then the term *Sjögren's syndrome* is used. Treatment of dry eyes consists primarily of the liberal use of artificial tears during the day and ointment at bedtime. Other modalities for more severe cases include occlusion of the puncta with thermal cautery or argon laser. Vitamin A, may offer some hope in patients with severe dry eyes.

Common retinal disorders

The eye is the window to the body and the observation of disorders of the living body. Many eye conditions are not seen on external examination but require the use of a direct or indirect ophthalmoscope to view the interior of the eye and in particular the retina and optic nerve. Some of these common retinal abnormalities are reviewed in this section. Short discussions will outline some of their causes and management. More detailed explanations may be found in standard ophthalmological textbooks.

RETINAL ARTERY OCCLUSION

Retinal artery occlusion is a true ocular catastrophe. If the central retinal artery is blocked by an embolus, the anterior nine layers of the retina undergo necrosis, resulting in total loss of light perception of that eye.

If the condition is seen within 30 minutes, there is a possibility of salvaging the eye by dilating the retinal arterioles to allow the embolus to move into the peripheral circulation.

The diagnosis is simple. There is a sudden and total loss of vision, the retina is gray (cloudy swelling of the retinal layers), and the blood vessels are attenuated and segmented. Ischemic changes make the entire nerve fiber layer of the retina gray. However, the macula does not have this layer, so it stands out, revealing the red blush from its choroidal vascular supply—hence, the quaint term for this sinister condition, the *cherry-red spot*. The usual prognosis is total and permanent loss of light perception for the involved eye.

RETINAL VEIN OCCLUSION

Central retinal vein occlusion is generally caused by a thrombus in a central retinal vein. Conditions that are associated with an increased risk of retinal vein occlusion include diabetes, hypertension, polycythemia, glaucoma, and any other condition that causes stasis of blood flow.

The patient may not be immediately aware of the onset of the condition, since there is no pain. The profound loss of vision may not be detected until the patient "discovers" it by rubbing or closing the good eye.

On ophthalmoscopic examination, the entire retina may be covered with superficial hemorrhages that appear flame-shaped. There may be scattered cotton-wool spots, which are microinfarcts of the retina. The retinal veins appear dilated and tortuous distal to the site of occlusion. The macula is usually edematous, and this leads to cystoid macular degeneration with a permanent loss of vision. If a branch of the vein is involved, only that sector through which it passes will be involved. Therefore in a branch vein occlusion the vision may not be affected. However, it is almost always the patients with visual loss that are seen in the ophthalmologist's office. The prognosis for visual recovery is significantly better with a branch vein occlusion than with a central vein occlusion.

The chances for visual recovery in a central retinal vein occlusion are generally poor. There is no effective treatment modality for restoring vision. The most dreaded complication is neovascular glaucoma, which can result in severe pain that may eventually be managed by enucleation. With ischemia there is proliferation of new vessels that can occur on the iris and extend over the trabecular meshwork. This can lead to obstruction of aqueous outflow and neovascular glaucoma.

Once the diagnosis is made of a central retinal vein occlusion, a fluorescein angiogram is usually performed to determine the degree of retinal ischemia. If there is significant ischemia, laser photocoagulation to all areas of the retina, that is, pan-retinal, can be performed. This is thought to destroy areas of ischemic retina that are probably responsible for producing a factor that leads to new blood vessel formation. The use of laser photocoagulation in selected cases has markedly decreased the incidence of neovascular glaucoma.

In branch vein occlusions, if there is macular involvement, vision will be decreased. Studies involving branch vein occlusions have shown that if vision has been decreased for more than 3 months and the fluorescein angiogram shows leakage of fluid in the macula, laser photocoagulation in a sector distribution can improve the visual prognosis. The risk of neovascular glaucoma is not generally a concern with branch vein occlusions.

Patients with venous occlusive disease should have a general medical evaluation to rule out diabetes, hypertension, or blood dyscrasias. The ophthalmologist must evaluate the nonaffected eye to rule out glaucoma, which is commonly associated with vein occlusions.

DIABETIC RETINOPATHY

Diabetes (see Chapter 6) may have a juvenile or adult onset. Generally, the incidence of diabetic complications increases with the duration of the disease. Complications may include systemic and ocular problems. Systemic complications include peripheral nerve disease, kidney disease, and vascular problems that can result in extremity pain and poor healing. Ocular problems tend to develop from no abnormalities to nonproliferative or background retinopathy and subsequently to proliferative retinopathy.

Background diabetic retinopathy includes the presence of microaneurysms (small vascular buds), dot and blot hemorrhages, and lipoid exudates from a serous leakage of the retinal vessels (Fig. 5-34). Preproliferative retinopathy includes cotton-wool spots, (microinfarcts of the retina), and intraretinal microvascular abnormalities (IRMA), which are capillaries within the retina that help supply ischemic areas. Proliferative retinopathy includes the presence of new vessel formation, that is, neovascularization, on the disc, the surface of the retina, or the iris. These fragile aberrant blood vessels are easily ruptured, causing recurrent retinal and vitreous hemorrhages. The neovascularization can contract to form a fibrovascular mass that can pull on the retina and lead to a retinal detachment. New vessel formation on the iris, with extension over the trabecular meshwork, can lead to neovascular glaucoma, which is difficult to treat.

Ocular treatment modalities for diabetes depend on the stage of the disease and the absence or presence of a variety of complications. If neovascularization is present, then pan-retinal photocoagulation is the treatment of choice. Approximately 2000 to 3000 burns are made with the argon laser. This destruction of ischemic retina is thought to decrease the secretion of the vasoproliferative factor by the retina. This in turn usually causes shrinkage and often resolution of the neovascularization. If the vision is decreased by macular edema, photocoagulation of leaking microaneurysms in the macular area has been shown to improve the visual prognosis. If the patient has a vitreous hem-

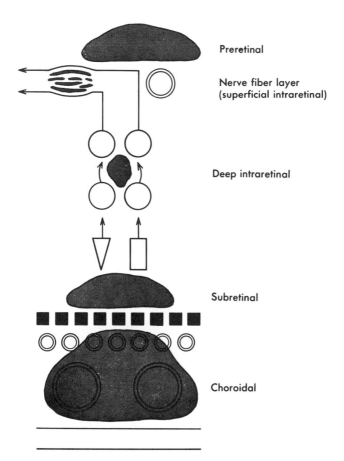

Preretinal

Nerve fiber layer
(superficial intraretinal)

Deep intraretinal

Subretinal

Choroidal

Fig. 5-34 Preretinal hemorrhage lying in front of retina. Note the location of intraretinal, subretinal, and choroidal hemorrhages.

orrhage that does not appear to be clearing after 1 to 3 months, or if there are fibrovascular bands producing a tractional retinal detachment, a vitrectomy is the surgical procedure of choice. The vitrectomy infusion suction and cutting instruments are introduced over the pars plana. The vitreous is removed and replaced with saline, and tractional bands are cut in the hope that the retina will fall back into its normal position.

The treatment of diabetes requires the entire coordinated effort of the ophthalmologist and the internist. Although the new technology has been beneficial, diabetic retinopathy remains one of the leading causes of blindness in North America.

RETINITIS PIGMENTOSA (Fig. 5-35)

Retinitis pigmentosa is a hereditary disorder that has a variable pattern of transmission. It can be passed on as a sex-linked trait or as an autosomal dominant or an autosomal recessive trait.

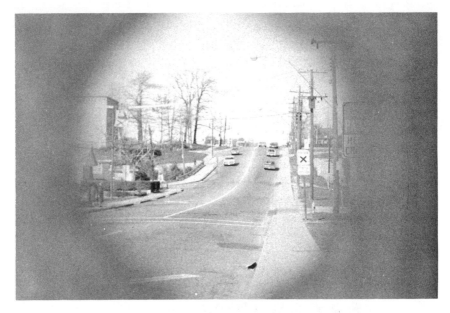

Fig. 5-35   Restricted peripheral visual field. The central field is clear.

It is a disease of the rods, so that the primary symptoms relate to a failure to see properly in dim illumination. The disease may be mild or may progress to cause total blindness, depending on the nature of the condition and its duration.

It is not inevitable that each case will develop and cause field loss that is constricting. Some cases of retinitis pigmentosa occur and then remain stationary for a lifetime.

The diagnosis is made by a visible inspection of the retina with the ophthalmoscope. The following findings are characteristic:

1. Bone spicule–like pigment debris in the midperiphery of the retina
2. Retinal vessel attenuation
3. Tubular visual fields
4. A waxy pallor of the disc

Occasionally a case will be found with typical symptoms but no retinal pigment dispersion. The electroretinogram (ERG) will show the depressed rod function, despite the absence of characteristic retinal changes.

Night blindness may also be caused by vitamin A deficiency, syphilis, and glaucoma.

At times, retinitis pigmentosa may occur with other disorders, including deafness, mental retardation, and, in the eye, cataracts, myopia, and glaucoma.

At this time, there is no specific treatment for this disease. It is important to elicit a genetic tree from the patient so that genetic counseling may be done. It is also imperative to follow the patient's progress. This is done to treat any complications that may occur and to ensure that the patient does not feel that the situation is hopeless. The handicap is great enough without gloomy predictions, which, in truth, may not be accurate. Many causes of retinitis pigmentosa are mild and either do not appear to progress or do so quite slowly. Naturally, people who develop the disease in their first decade are worse off than those people who seem to develop retinitis pigmentosa in their forties or fifties.

In many states and provinces, there are retinitis pigmentosa foundations. Patients should be directed to these groups for counseling, assurance, and a line to new therapies.

RETINOPATHY OF PREMATURITY

Retinopathy of prematurity is a proliferative vascular disease occurring in premature infants exposed to high concentrations of oxygen soon after birth. The fibrovascular proliferation can lead to retinal detachment or a white retrolental membrane (behind the lens of the eye). The disease is usually bilateral and, in severe cases, will cause blindness.

Prevention of this disease is of utmost importance. The pediatrician should try to use the lowest oxygen level that is compatible with good neonatal care. An eye examination should be done at the time of discharge from the hospital on all premature infants who received significant oxygen therapy. Careful follow-up examinations should be done to rule out any fibrovascular proliferation. Treatment of retinopathy of prematurity may include observation for spontaneous regression, cryosurgery, vitrectomy, or retinal detachment surgery.

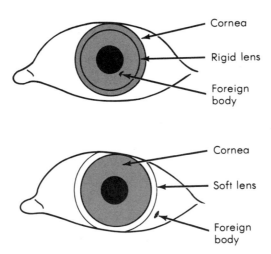

Fig. 5-36 The rigid lens permits foreign particles to enter under the lens, whereas the soft lens tends to prevent the tracking of foreign bodies under it by its scleral impingement and minimum movement. (From Stein HA and Slatt BJ: Fitting guide for rigid and soft contact lenses, a practical approach, ed 2, St Louis, 1984, The CV Mosby Co.)

RETINAL BREAKS

Retinal breaks may take the form of holes or tears. A retinal hole is often the result of an atrophic process that leads to a through-and-through defect of the retina. If it occurs in the macula, it causes a permanent loss of vision to 20/200 or less. A different type of hole and a tear can be produced when a detaching vitreous pulls off a small piece of retina. If the operculum, or everting lip of retinal tissue, is still attached to the retina, a retinal tear is produced. If the operculum is free from the retina, a hole is produced.

Most retinal tears and holes occur in the periphery of the retina, and detection requires a fully dilated pupil and visualization with an indirect ophthalmoscope. Sometimes hemorrhage may occur as a sudden shower. All retinal tears in which the retina is not detached should be sealed by the laser beam to prevent the possible entry of lique-fied vitreous through the tear and between the pigment epithelium and the retina. The use of the laser in this manner will usually prevent the retina from detaching. All retinal holes in which the patient has recently exhibited symptoms of flashing lights or floaters should be treated with laser photocoagulation.

CENTRAL SEROUS CHORIORETINOPATHY

This is a type of retinal detachment that involves the macula but is unassociated with a retinal tear or hole. Serous detachment of the macula is more common in males than in females, and typically occurs in patients 25 to 50 years of age. There appears to be strong association between stress and the development of this disorder.

The symptoms are often highly characteristic. The patient not only complains of blurred vision but will commonly describe distortion of vision with loss of color perception. Objects often appear curved, darker in color, and smaller.

Fluorescein angiography typically shows a leakage point in which fluid passes from the choroid, through a defect in the pigment epithelium, to a location beneath the retina. Most cases clear spontaneously and therefore require no specific therapy. Treatment may be indicated in cases that have prolonged visual loss or show degenerative changes in the retina. Treatment is with laser photocoagulation to seal the defect in the pigment epithelium.

CHANGES IN THE RETINA FROM CONCUSSION
Commotio retinae (Berlin's "edema")

A blow to the front of the eye can cause a disalignment of the outer segments of the photoreceptors. The involved retina is not edematous. It has a whitish appearance resulting from structural changes of the photoreceptors. With time the whitish appearance resolves and some mild pigmentary changes of the retina can be seen ophthalmoscopically. If the macula is affected, a permanent reduction in vision can occur.

Retinal hemorrhages

Retinal hemorrhages may be in front of the retina (preretinal), under the retina (subretinal), or within the retina (intraretinal).

Birth injury is a common cause of traumatic retinal hemorrhage of the newborn.

Retinal detachment

Although retinal detachment is uncommon, patients with retinal injury must be watched because the detachment can occur months or even years after the injury.

FOREIGN BODY IN THE EYE

The degree of damage depends on the mechanical disruption of tissue, as well as the chemical injury specific to a type of metal within the eye.

A foreign body composed of relatively pure copper (greater than 90%) can cause a massive purulent inflammation. Copper in a concentration of 70% to 90% will cause chalcosis, with the deposition of copper in intraocular structures possibly leading to cataracts and glaucoma. If the foreign body is an alloy of copper in a concentration of less than 70%, it will rarely cause any intraocular problems.

Gold, silver, platinum, aluminum, and glass are chemically inert and do damage only by disruption of the tissues.

A retained iron foreign body can cause siderosis bulbi. In the retina, it destroys the sensory elements and can cause a profound loss of vision indicated by a flat or extinguished ERG. The entire retina eventually becomes saturated with iron. The trabecular meshwork can also be affected, which can result in glaucoma. These changes can be observed for months to years after the accident. If the foreign body is removed at an early stage, the entire process of siderosis bulbi may be prevented.

Iron injuries are common. Fortunately, metallic foreign bodies are magnetic. This makes removal easier, because the magnetic particle can be drawn out of the eye with relative ease.

Most retained ocular foreign bodies are a result of industrial accidents. The best treatment is prevention, which means advocating safety glasses. The most impregnable lens is made of polycarbonate, which will withstand the force of a bullet.

ECLIPSE BURNS OF THE RETINA

Following an exposure of minutes, or even seconds, to an eclipse, the macular area may be burned by the infrared rays of the sun. Once a hole is made in the macula from an eclipse burn, the results are permanent.

There is no absolutely safe way to protect children against such mishaps. The best treatment is prevention. Even when proper dense filters are recommended for observing an eclipse, there is no guarantee of patient compliance, especially with young children.

SENILE MACULAR DEGENERATION

There are a great variety of clinical conditions that are labeled *senile macular degeneration*. The clinical findings that may be present include:

1. *Absent foveal reflex.* This is the most subtle of changes. The architecture of the fovea is slightly altered so that the reflex of the foveal pit is not seen.
2. *Pigment mottling.* These macular changes are caused by scattered areas of clumping and atrophy of the pigment epithelium.
3. *Drusen.* These are small, yellowish white lesions located between the retinal

pigment epithelium and Bruch's membrane. They are a common aging change and a predisposing factor of splitting of Bruch's membrane, which can lead to neovascularization from the choroid.

4. *Subretinal neovascularization.* These new vessels can leak serum or blood and cause a serous or hemorrhagic detachment of the pigment epithelium, resulting in a dramatic decrease in vision. When the blood has not broken through the retina, it may appear as a black mass and simulate a malignant melanoma. If these new vessels are detected early and confirmed with a fluorescein angiogram, laser treatment can be employed in an attempt to destroy the abnormal vessels and prevent subsequent leakage.

5. *Disciform degeneration of the macula.* If serum or blood leaks into the macula, the healing process can lead to gliosis, which leaves a flat grayish white scar. This scar results in permanent loss of central vision, whereas the peripheral field of vision is left intact. Degenerative changes can also occur if the pigment epithelium undergoes atrophy, which leads to death of the photoreceptors and a decrease in vision.

Senile macular degeneration is one of the most common causes of loss of vision in the elderly. Generally, for most patients, no specific remedy can be offered. However, for a small percentage of patients, the laser can be used to coagulate subretinal neovascularization. This can prevent or slow down the degenerative process. Since most elderly people with bilateral disciform degeneration have a visual acuity often reduced to 20/200 or less, visual aids are necessary to enable them to read.

OCULAR MANIFESTATIONS OF COMMON SYSTEMIC DISEASES
Hypertension

Patients with high blood pressure or hypertension (see Chapter 6) are commonly diagnosed by the ophthalmologist.

In the early phase of the disease, the only manifestation may be an attenuation of the retinal arterioles. This narrowing may be uniform, as found in older people, or focal, which may occur in a younger person.

In the elderly, the changes may be mild as the retinal vessels become thicker with a dulling of the light reflexes on the retinal arteriole surface. At the area of crossings, the retinal arterioles may compress the underlying veins and cause banking or arteriovenous nicking of the underlying blood column.

Younger patients with severe hypertension may display a florid type of retinopathy with flame-shaped hemorrhages, exudates, cotton-wool spots, and marked narrowing of the retinal arterioles.

The most ominous sign is edema, or swelling, of the optic disc. Patients with this symptom have an extremely poor survival rate.

Sickle cell disease

Sickle cell hemoglobinopathies are most common in black people. The disorder is hereditary. The normal hemoglobin is replaced by the sickle hemoglobin in the red cell.

Retinal changes are common in the severe form of the disease. These include retinal arteriole occlusions, neovascular budding of vessels on the surface of the retina, leading to retinal and vitreous hemorrhages, and preretinal membranes. Comma-shaped capillaries in the conjunctiva are part of the general vascular pattern.

Thyroid disorders

Ocular disease can be seen in patients with hyperthyroidism (excessive thyroid activity), hypothyroidism (depressed thyroid activity), and even euthyroidism (normal thyroid function after successful treatment for hyperthyroidism).

Hyperthyroid people tend to have a rapid pulse, shortness of breath, and a loss of weight. Hypothyroid people show a deceleration of activity and may be dull mentally, with a low voice, reduced pulse rate, dry skin, and a gain in weight.

Patients with a thyroid disorder and specific eye findings have a condition referred to as Graves' disease. The etiologic factors of this condition are thought to be immunologic. A variety of tests can be employed for diagnosis of the thyroid condition: serum thyroxine, T_3 resin uptake, thyroid autoantibodies, thyrotropin-releasing hormone (TRH), and T_3 assay.

The ocular manifestations of Graves' disease are discussed in Chapter 6, pp. 152-155. Management of Graves' disease involves both the internist, to treat and manage the thyroid condition, and the ophthalmologist, to deal with the ocular complications. Guanethidine eyedrops, 10%, are often helpful in reducing the lid retraction, which is cosmetically disfiguring. The lid retraction can also be aided surgically by cutting Müller's muscle and a section of the levator palpebrae superioris.

Exposure keratitis can be managed by the liberal use of lubrication in the form of artificial tears and ointment. Therapy is indicated if the orbital congestion causes a decrease in either color vision or central vision, or a defect on visual field testing. Therapy may consist of systemic steroids, orbital radiation, or an orbital decompression (removing a wall of the orbit) to reduce the severe orbital pressure. If double vision results, muscle surgery can be used to relax the muscles and align the eyes.

INFECTIOUS DISEASES OF THE RETINA AND CHOROID
Toxoplasmosis (see Fig. 9-18)

Toxoplasma gondii is a protozoan parasite that can cause retinochoroiditis, especially in the congenital form. The congenital disease is a result of intrauterine infection. This disease is more severe because it is bilateral, and inflammatory deposits may also appear in the brain. The macular region is affected most commonly so that this infection results in considerable visual loss. (See Chapter 6, pp. 159-160, for a further discussion.)

In the active stage, the affected retina looks gray and edematous with overlying vitreous haze. In the healed phase, there is chorioretinal atrophy so that a white punched-out area is visible, surrounded by a fringe of pigment.

The diagnosis of toxoplasmosis is basically a clinical one, since ocular cultures cannot be taken. A variety of blood tests, however, can be done to document whether the patient has ever been exposed to toxoplasmosis. The problem inherent in the results is that 50% of the population has been exposed to this organism; hence the only valuable result is a negative blood test. Active infection with involvement of, or close to, the optic disc or macula should be aggressively treated with systemic antibiotics. These may include sulfadiazine, pyrimethamine, or clindamycin.

Histoplasmosis

Histoplasma capsulatum is a fungus that is commonly responsible for significant ocular morbidity. The infection is most prevalent in certain river valleys in the zone from 45 degrees north latitude to 45 degrees south latitude. In the United States, people living in the Mississippi and Ohio River Valley areas are most commonly affected. The clinical features may include "punched-out" chorioretinal scars, peripapillary scarring, and subretinal neovascular membranes. This last condition can lead to exudates and hemorrhages in a subretinal macular location, which can result in a permanent decrease in vision. If the new vessels are detected early, laser photocoagulation may be employed to improve the visual prognosis.

MALIGNANT MELANOMA

The tumor, although rare, is the most common malignant neoplasm found in the eye. These lesions are 15 times more prevalent in whites than in blacks, are more common in males than in females, and are often detected in the fifth and sixth decades of life.

Clinical symptoms may be absent unless the macula is involved with a resultant decrease in vision, or if there is an overlying retinal detachment with a field loss. The tumor appears as a greenish brown choroidal mass that in an advanced state may assume a mushroom shape if the tumor breaks through Bruch's membrane.

A variety of treatment modalities can be offered. The technique used depends on the size of the lesion. For small tumors, usually less than 1 cm in size, observation with sequential fundus photographs to detect growth may be the practice of choice. For larger tumors, management is usually a choice between the use of radioactive plaques (attached to the globe over the tumor site) and enucleation. This is an area of great controversy, because studies have shown an increase in mortality following enucleation and suggest that tumor shedding may occur during removal of the eye. Long-term results of radiation therapy are not well known. Because of these uncertainties, the patient and the clinician are often faced with a difficult decision regarding the most appropriate management. A new technique of resecting only the tumor and leaving the remainder of the eye may prove to be therapeutically efficacious.

The prognosis with and without treatment cannot be given with certainty. Even after enucleations, spread of the tumor has been reported 20 years after the diagnosis has been made. The tumor has a predilection to metastasize to the liver, the skin, and bone. When the tumor has spread outside of the eye, the survival rate is usually less than 1 year. New developments in the field of immunology, in which cells are created to attack specific tumor cells, may eventually lead to an improvement in survival.

6 Common systemic disorders affecting the eye

The ocular examination may provide important clues to the systemic well-being of an individual. The recognition of specific ocular signs can often be helpful in establishing a systemic diagnosis and/or determining its severity. A variety of systemic disorders will be discussed in this chapter; many of these are common, but some are rare, with important diagnostic features.

DIABETES

Diabetes is a complex metabolic disorder manifested by excretion of a large volume of sugared urine, loss of weight, abnormal thirst, and fatigue. It is usually genetically determined and is a leading causes of blindness in North America. The cause of diabetes is unknown, but the basic defect appears to be a relative or absolute lack of insulin.

Diabetes can lead to both ocular and systemic complications. The systemic manifestations include, most importantly, disease of the kidneys, peripheral nervous system, and blood vessels.

The incidence of diabetic retinopathy increases with the duration of diabetes. Juvenile diabetics who have had diabetes for 5 years or less show no evidence of diabetic retinopathy. However, 25% will have diabetic retinopathy if the diabetes has been present for 5 to 10 years. Of patients who have had diabetes for longer than 10 years, 71% will have diabetic retinopathy. After 30 years, 90% will have diabetic retinopathy and one third of these will have proliferative retinopathy.

Diabetic eye disease can be classified into three general categories: background, preproliferative, and proliferative diabetic retinopathy.

Background diabetic retinopathy. Background diabetic retinopathy is characterized by microaneurysms, hard exudates, and dot, blot, or splinter hemorrhages. The microaneurysms are outpouchings from the walls of the capillaries. These areas of vascular dilation are in areas of pericytes dropout. Hard exudates are derived from the serum and appear as yellow deposits in the outer plexiform layer of the retina. Dot or blot hemorrhages are round or oval and occur in the inner nuclear layer or outer plexiform layer.

Flame- or splinter-shaped hemorrhages are superficial and occur in the nerve fiber bundles.

Preproliferative diabetic retinopathy. Preproliferative diabetic retinopathy is characterized by cotton-wool spots and intraretinal microvascular abnormalities (IRMA). The cotton-wool spots appear as white retinal patches and are secondary to ischemic damage to the nerve fiber layer of the retina. IRMA, which are also secondary to hypoxia, may be difficult to differentiate from new vessel formation. With the technique of fluorescein angiography the new vessels leak fluorescein and the vessels of IRMA do not.

Proliferative diabetic retinopathy. Proliferative diabetic retinopathy is manifested by neovascularization (Fig. 6-1), which may occur on the disc or retina. This new vessel growth is probably a vascular response to a hypoxic retinal environment. These fragile vessels can easily rupture and result in a preretinal hemorrhage, which is located beneath the internal limiting membrane of the retina or a vitreous hemorrhage. The neovascularization is usually accompanied by a fibrous component that can result in shrinkage and lead to a retinal detachment. Occasionally the neovascularization can affect the iris and the trabecular meshwork and lead to obstruction of aqueous humor outflow, which results in a condition called *neovascular glaucoma.*

Laser photocoagulation is the most commonly used treatment for diabetic retinopathy. It may be used to treat macular edema and the proliferative phase of the disease. In macular edema the fluorescein angiogram will demonstrate the microaneurysms and other leakage points, which, if the process is not too diffuse, can be directly photocoagulated. If the leakage is diffuse, photocoagulation can be performed in a grid pattern. In proliferative retinopathy, the technique of panretinal photocoagulation is used. In this procedure more than 1500 laser burns are scattered over the retina; if done early in the process of the disease, this procedure may result in regression of the neovascularization and preservation of vision.

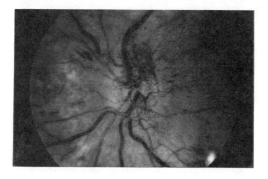

Fig. 6-1   Neovascularization of the disc in a patient with diabetes mellitus. (From Stein H, Slatt B, and Stein R: Ophthalmic Terminology, ed 2, St Louis, The CV Mosby Co, 1987.)

HYPERTENSION

Hypertension is associated with a large increase in morbidity and mortality from various causes. Although there is no sharp dividing line between normal and elevated blood pressure, an adult is considered by many to be hypertensive if arterial pressure is 160/95 mm Hg or higher. Of the adult population in North America, 15% to 20% have values at or above this range. Hypertension results in an increased risk of premature death and vascular disease involving the eyes, brain, heart, and kidneys.

Hypertension affects all the blood vessels in the body, but those in the eyes are most readily observable. A variety of vascular and retinal changes can be noted in hypertension. These will be discussed next.

Generalized narrowing. Elevation of blood pressure for a prolonged period results in narrowing or attenuation of the arterioles. A definite relationship exists between the diastolic pressure and these arteriole changes. Clinically, the size of the artery to the vein can be compared. Normally the ratio is 2:3; that is, the artery is two thirds the size of the vein. With narrowing of the arteriole the ratio may decrease to 1:3.

Sclerosis of the arterioles. Arteriosclerosis occurs when the blood pressure remains elevated. Thickening of the blood vessel wall occurs as a compensatory mechanism. Clinically, a change in the light reflex can be observed. The light reflex from the vessel decreases with progression of the sclerosis. It can be described as having a "copper wire" appearance. With progressive sclerosis, the vessel becomes whitish and is likened to a silver wire.

Focal constriction. Focal constriction is a localized, symmetrical narrowing of the arterioles. The arteriole abruptly changes from a relatively normal caliber to constricted and then to normal. The segments often vary in number, length, and location. Focal constriction is usually associated with a severely elevated diastolic pressure, often greater than 110 mm Hg.

Crossing changes. Crossing changes occur in the artery and vein over a period of years. These changes occur most commonly in hypertensive individuals or may be a manifestation of aging without elevated blood pressure. Compression or nicking of the vein by the arteriole (Gunn's sign) and a change in the course of the vein under the artery (Salus's sign) can be observed clinically.

Hemorrhages. The hemorrhages in hypertension are usually located in the nerve fiber layer and are characterized by a splinter or flame shape.

Cotton-wool spots. Infarcts to the nerve fiber layer of the retina produce cotton-wool spots. These often clear spontaneously over a period of several weeks. Histologically there remains a focal area of degeneration of an axon called a *cytoid body.*

Edema residues. Hard or waxy exudates represent lipid-rich collections of plasma deposited in the retina. The residues appear as yellowish-white deposits in the deep layers of the retina. These deposits are most common in the posterior pole. In the macula the deposits may form a "macular star."

Papilledema. The finding of papilledema represents the severe form of hypertension. The disc edema results from ischemia caused by arteriolar occlusion and leakage of individual vessels.

Clinical findings

The eye findings in hypertension can be expressed according to a grading system developed by Keith, Wagener, and Baker of the Mayo Clinic. Four grades of hypertensive retinopathy are considered:

- Grade 1 consists of mild narrowing and sclerosis of the retinal vessels.
- Grade 2 changes consist of more marked retinal vessel changes with localized or generalized arteriolar narrowing and retinal arteriovenous crossing phenomena.
- Grade 3 comprises grade 2 plus retinopathy. This may include retinal hemorrhages, cotton-wool spots, and exudates (Fig. 6-2). The mean life expectancy for patients in this category is less than 3 years.
- Grade 4 hypertensive retinopathy consists of grade 3 findings plus papilledema and is seen only in severe cases of hypertension. The mean life expectancy for these patients is less than 1 year.

GRAVES' DISEASE

Graves' disease is characterized by specific ocular features in a patient who usually has a hyperthyroid condition. The thyroid dysfunction and the ophthalmopathy may not occur at the same time. The exact cause of Graves' disease is unknown; however, there is evidence that this is an immune disease. Immune complexes, lympocytes, plasma cells, and mass cells have been identified within the extraocular muscles. In a high percentage of patients circulating antibodies to ocular muscles can be detected.

A variety of ocular signs are seen in thyroid-related eye disease; these are discussed next.

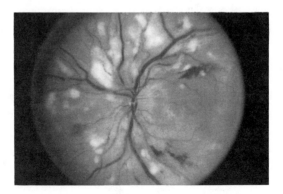

Fig. 6-2 Advanced hypertensive retinopathy (grade 3) with narrowed arterioles, scattered hemorrhages, and cotton-wool spots. (Courtesy Department of Ophthalmology, Mayo Clinic.) (From Stein H, Slatt B, and Stein R: Ophthalmic Terminology, ed 2, St Louis, The CV Mosby Co, 1987.)

Lid retraction. Lid retraction may occur of the upper and/or lower lids. This may produce scleral show and hence the characteristic "startled" appearance.

Lid lag. Lid lag is demonstrated by having the patient look from upgaze to downgaze and noting the relative lag of the lid position to the movement of the globe.

Eyelid edema. Eyelid edema may be an early sign of Graves' disease.

Chemosis. Edema (chemosis) of the conjunctiva and injection over the rectus muscles.

Proptosis. Exophthalmos or proptosis (protrusion of the eye) (Fig. 6-3) may be seen. In Graves' disease swelling of the retrobulbar tissues within the confines of a bony orbit results in the eye being pushed forward. The extent of protrusion of the eye is measured with the exophthalmometer (Fig. 6-4). Thyroid dysfunction is the most common cause of unilateral or bilateral proptosis in the adult.

Restriction of ocular motility. Restriction occurs because of the inability of the fibrotic eye muscles to relax. Involvement is most common in decreasing order of fre-

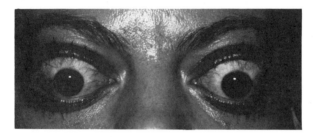

Fig. 6-3 Thyroid exophthalmos. A patient with Graves' disease who demonstrates characteristic signs of lid retraction and proptosis. (Courtesy Brian Younge, MD, Department of Ophthalmology, Mayo Clinic; from Stein H, Slatt B, and Stein R: Ophthalmic Terminology, ed 2, St Louis, The CV Mosby Co, 1987.)

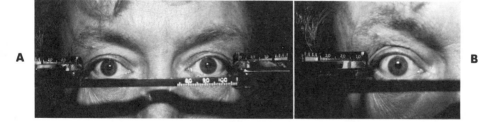

Fig. 6-4 **A,** The Hertel exophthalmometer is used to measure the amount of proptosis. **B,** A higher magnification view demonstrates the ease in which proptosis can be measured with the exophthalmometer. (Courtesy Brian Younge, MD, Department of Ophthalmology, Mayo Clinic; from Stein H, Slatt B, and Stein R: Ophthalmic Terminology, ed 2, St Louis, The CV Mosby Co, 1987.)

quency of the inferior rectus, medial rectus, superior rectus, and lateral rectus. This restriction in eye movement can be differentiated from a muscle weakness problem by checking the intraocular pressure when the patient looks straight ahead, compared with upgaze. In Graves' disease the tight extraocular muscles press on the globe in upgaze, and the intraocular pressure increases, unlike that seen with a nonrestrictive problem. Another means is by the technique of forced ductions, in which a drop of anesthetic is placed onto the eye and then forceps are used to grasp the globe and move it. In Graves' disease the tethered extraocular muscles prevent the free movement of the globe.

Corneal complications. Keratitis may result secondary to drying of the ocular surface (Fig. 6-5). This has been attributed to upper lid retraction, exophthalmos, and a decreased blink rate.

Optic neuropathy. Visual loss can result from optic nerve compression by the surrounding swollen orbital tissues. The optic neuropathy can occur early in the disease course with only mild or no proptosis. Evaluation of optic nerve dysfunction may include an assessment of an afferent pupillary defect and color vision testing.

The diagnosis of Graves' disease is confirmed with the clinical features as described and a computed tomographic (CT) scan (Fig. 6-6) that shows enlargement of the extraocular muscles. The patient usually has a hyperthyroid condition and shows evidence of an enlarged thyroid gland (goiter), fine tremor, increased nervousness, palpitations, weight loss with increased appetite, warm skin, and tachycardia at rest.

Graves' ophthalmopathy may also be associated with hypothyroidism. Clinical indicators include weight gain with decreased appetite, bradycardia, and lethargy.

The ophthalmopathy may also be associated with a euthyroid state. In testing for euthyroid Graves' disease, the following investigations should be undertaken. The patient should be tested initially for triiodothyronine (T_3) and thyroxine (T_4) resin uptake to exclude the possibility of active thyroid disease. If this test is normal, a serum T_3 test is performed. If the results of this test are normal, a thyrotropin-releasing hormone (TRH) test is done. This shows normal release of thyroid-stimulating hormone (TSH). If the results of this test are normal, one can make the diagnosis of euthyroid Graves' disease.

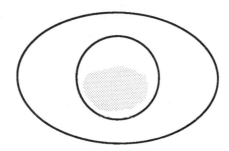

Fig. 6-5 Exposure keratopathy in Graves' disease.

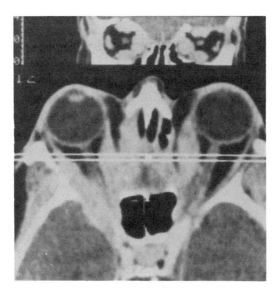

Fig. 6-6 Computed tomographic scan showing thickened extraocular muscles characteristic of Graves' disease. *Top,* a coronal scan: superior-inferior cut; *Bottom,* a transaxial scan: anterior-posterior cut. (From Brian Younge, MD, Department of Ophthalmology, Mayo Clinic; from Stein H, Slatt B, and Stein R: Ophthalmic Terminology, ed 2, St Louis, The CV Mosby Co, 1987.)

Treatment of Graves' disease involves attention to the ophthalmopathy and to the hyperthyroidism. Lubrication and ointment can be used for corneal exposure. Systemic steroids, radiation, or both can be used to decrease the marked congestion. A variety of surgical procedures can be performed to decompress the orbits so as to allow more room for the swollen tissues. A Krönlein procedure is a lateral approach to decompressing the orbit. A transantral decompression is an inferior approach that allows some bulging of the orbital tissues in the maxillary sinus. Decompression procedures are used when the optic nerve is compressed and vision is threatened. If the disease has stabilized, muscle surgery and lid surgery can be performed. The muscle surgery is used to relax the tight fibrotic muscles to improve motility and alleviate diplopia. Lid surgery can improve the cosmetic appearance by reducing the retraction by recessing Müller's muscle and if necessary the levator palpebras superioris.

Radioactive iodine can be used to manage the hyperthyroidism by destroying the thyroid tissue. This treatment is simple and involves no surgical complications or hospitalization. The major difficulty is the onset of hypothyroidism after therapy, which may be present in 40% to 80% of patients after 10 years. A subtotal thyroidectomy, a surgical procedure that removes the majority of the thyroid gland, can also be used in the management of hyperthyroidism.

SARCOIDOSIS

Sarcoidosis is an idiopathic granulomatous disease with a variety of systemic and ocular features. Sarcoid granulomas may form in almost any organ, producing varying degrees

Table 6-1   Systemic involvement in sarcoidosis

Involved organ	Rate of occurrence (%)
Intrathoracic	
Hilar lymphadenopathy	70.0
Lung parenchyma	53.0
Extrathoracic	
Ocular	38.0
Peripheral lymphadenopathy	27.8
Cutaneous	22.9
Hepatomegaly	22.0
Splenomegaly	13.0
Central nervous system	8.7
Musculoskeletal	7.2
Parotid	5.8
Cardiac	3.2
Other	5.1

Table 6-2   Ophthalmic sarcoidosis

Abnormality	Rate of occurrence (%)
Anterior segment	84.7
Chronic uveitis	52.5
Iris nodules	11.4
Acute iritis	14.9
Cataracts	8.4
Conjunctival lesion	6.9
Band keratopathy	4.5
Interstitial keratitis	1.0
Posterior segment disease	25.3
Chorioretinitis	10.9
Periphlebitis	10.4
Chorioretinal nodules	5.5
Vitreous cells	3.0
Vitreous hemorrhage	1.5
Retinal neovascularization	1.5
Orbital and other disease	26.2
Lacrimal gland	15.8
Optic nerve	7.4
Motility	2.0
Orbital granuloma	1.0

From Obenauf CD, Shaw HE, Sydnor CF, et al: Sarcoidosis and its ophthalmic manifestations. Am J Ophthalmol 1978;86:648-655.

of inflammation and dysfunction (Tables 6-1 and 6-2). The lungs, eyes, and skin are most commonly involved. There is a predilection for an intrathoracic hilar lymphadenopathy, with or without pulmonary infiltrates or fibrosis. Other sites of granuloma formation include the spleen, kidneys, liver, muscles, bones, and the central and peripheral nervous system.

Ocular involvement in sarcoidosis may include the following manifestations.

Eyelid nodules. Granulomatous nodules of the eyelids may be the only ophthalmic manifestation.

Conjunctival nodules. Inflammation of the conjunctiva can result in granulomatous nodules (Fig. 6-7).

Anterior uveitis. Anterior uveitis is usually bilateral and recurrent and may become chronic. Nodules caused by granulomas commonly develop on the pupillary border of the iris (Koeppe's nodules) or in the iris stroma (Busacca's nodules). The uveitis is often severe and may be complicated by peripheral anterior synechiae, glaucoma, cataract, and calcific band keratopathy.

Posterior segment involvement. The posterior segment is involved in approximately 25% of patients with ocular sarcoidosis. The findings may include cystoid macular edema, aggregates of inflammatory cells around retinal veins (candlewax drippings), retinal hemorrhages, neovascularization, and choroidal granulomas. In addition, the optic nerve may be affected. This may be manifested as edema, atrophy, or granulomas of the optic nerve.

Management

A histopathologic diagnosis is necessary before oral steroid therapy is initiated for the systemic complications. The sarcoid granuloma contains macrophages, epithelioid cells, T and B lymphocytes, and multinucleated giant cells. Conjunctival biopsies yield positive results in 30% to 50% of cases in which follicles are seen. If the conjunctiva appears normal, the incidence of a positive biopsy is only 10%. A transbronchial lung biopsy using a flexible fiberoptic bronchoscope may be necessary.

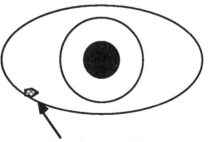

Sarcoid nodule of the inferior conjunctiva

Fig. 6-7 Sarcoidosis may present in the eye with a conjunctival nodule. A conjunctival biopsy is an easy approach to making a histopathologic diagnosis.

Angiotensin-converting enzyme (ACE) is derived from epithelioid cells and other monocytes. Although not diagnostic of sarcoidosis, the serum ACE level may be useful in monitoring a patient's clinical course as it correlates with disease activity.

Management of ocular involvement in sarcoidosis is usually with topical steroids in conjunction with long-acting cycloplegics. If the posterior aspect of the eye is involved, this usually correlates with significant systemic disease, and oral steroids are usually indicated.

The majority of sarcoid patients do not require systemic therapy, and about two thirds recover completely with essentially no sequelae. Overall mortality for sarcoidosis is less than 5%. Pulmonary insufficiency is the most common cause of death.

COLLAGEN VASCULAR DISEASES

Collagen vascular diseases not uncommonly have ocular manifestations. A variety of diseases and their potential ocular complications are discussed next.

Ankylosing spondylitis. Anterior uveitis occurs in about one third of patients with ankylosing spondylitis. There is a high incidence of recurrence of the uveitis. The uveitis may precede the diagnosis of ankylosing spondylitis. Treatment is with topical steroids and cycloplegics.

Reiter's syndrome. Reiter's syndrome is classically characterized by the triad of arthritis, conjunctivitis, and urethritis. The pathogenesis of RS is not clear; however, the disease appears to occur in patients with a genetic predisposition and who are exposed to certain microorganisms. Conjunctivitis is the most common ocular manifestation. The infection is usually mild and associated with a mucopurulent discharge. Attempts to isolate organisms from the conjunctiva have been unsuccessful. The second most common manifestation is an acute iridocyclitis. Other potential complications include episcleritis, scleritis, and posterior uveitis.

Adult rheumatoid arthritis. Rheumatoid arthritis is a chronic, inflammatory, multisystem disease of unknown cause that is characterized by a polyarthropathy. Ocular features may include keratitis sicca (dry eyes), episcleritis, scleritis, and peripheral corneal melting.

Juvenile rheumatoid arthritis. Juvenile rheumatoid arthritis is potentially both a crippling and a blinding disease. The ocular features may consist of a chronic anterior uveitis, glaucoma, and calcific band keratopathy.

Wegener's disease. Wegener's disease is characterized by a necrotizing granulomatous vasculitis, which can involve multiple organ systems, including the respiratory tract, the kidneys, and the eyes. Ocular involvement may include a progressive marginal ulcerative keratitis, scleritis, episcleritis, and conjunctival inflammation.

LEUKEMIAS

Approximately 50% of patients with leukemia will have ocular involvement. The ocular complications are more common with the acute leukemias, such as myelogenous, monocytic, or acute lymphocytic leukemia.

Iris/anterior chamber. Accumulation of tumor cells may form iris nodules. Tumor cells may collect in the anterior chamber and simulate a hypopyon. The trabecular meshwork may be infiltrated, resulting in glaucoma.

Retina. Retinal complications may include cotton-wool spots, hemorrhages, perivascular sheathing, and tortuous veins. In addition, preretinal and vitreous hemorrhages may result.

Optic nerve. Infiltration of the optic disc by leukemic cells will produce disc swelling. This process is usually unilateral and must be differentiated from papilledema, which is bilateral.

ACQUIRED IMMUNODEFICIENCY SYNDROME (AIDS)

There are a variety of ocular complications of AIDS. Occasionally the patient is initially seen because of an ocular complaint.

Cytomegalovirus (CMV) retinitis. The retina may show intraretinal hemorrhages and cotton-wool spots. CMV retinitis is the most common ocular feature of AIDS; it is seen in approximately one third of patients.

Kaposi's sarcoma. Kaposi's sarcoma is a vascularized lesion that may occur on the lid or conjunctiva, as well as on other body regions. An excisional biopsy is indicated.

Herpes zoster ophthalmicus (HZO). In patients who have HZO in an atypical age-group (20 to 45 years), one should suspect AIDS. The clinical features and disease course is more severe in immunocompromised patients.

Other infections. Other opportunistic infections may occur: toxoplasmosis, cryptococcus, atypical mycobacterial infection, and herpes simplex retinitis.

Infectious disease

PHARYNGOCONJUNCTIVAL FEVER (PCF)

Infection with a few specific types of adenoviruses (for example, types 3 or 7) may cause a condition manifested by a sore throat, fever, and a red eye. The disease predominates in children and young adults. The eye findings are typically that of a conjunctivitis with a watery discharge and occasional corneal involvement. The disease will often affect both eyes and is highly contagious. PCF usually runs its own course over several weeks. No specific treatment is indicated and no permanent eye damage results.

TOXOPLASMOSIS

Toxoplasmosis (see Fig. 9-18) is caused by the parasite *Toxoplasma gondii.* Infection may be either congenital or acquired (raw meat, cat feces). Systemic manifestations are more common in the congenital form and may include intracranial calcification, convulsions, and mental retardation.

Most cases of acquired systemic toxoplasmosis are subclinical in nature. The lymphadenopathic form is the most common clinical type. There are no symptoms, but there is a localized lymphadenopathy. It is responsible for approximately 15% of unexplained lymphadenopathies. Other clinical manifestations of acquired toxoplasmosis include encephalitis, polymyositis, pneumonitis, and psychiatric disturbances. Ocular disease in the congenital and acquired forms may be manifested by the following.

Retinochoroiditis. Retinochoroiditis, an infection of the retina and adjacent choroid, is the ocular counterpart of central nervous system involvement by *T. gondii.* The parasite may remain dormant in a cystic stage for years. Recurrent active retinitis is thought to be caused by rupture of cysts, which produces areas of acute inflammation. The retinal lesions are characterized by yellow-white inflammatory areas that are often adjacent to an old scar (Fig. 6-8).

Iridocyclitis. Iridocyclitis, an inflammatory reaction, is probably produced by immune-mediated mechanisms, since no toxoplasma organisms have ever been found in the anterior part of the eye.

Disc edema. Disc edema may be a papillitis from optic nerve involvement or papilledema from ruptured cerebral cysts, producing raised intracranial pressure.

Diagnosis is confirmed by the indirect-fluorescent antibody test, which measures serum antibodies that are directed against the toxoplasma organism.

Treatment is indicated if the inflammatory process threatens the macula or optic nerve. Pyrimethamine and sulfadiazine are the most commonly used antibiotics. Clindamycin, which has been evaluated on an experimental basis, has shown favorable preliminary results.

TOXOCARIASIS

Toxocariasis is caused by the parasite *Toxocara canis.* The disease is usually acquired by children who ingest the *Toxocara* eggs that have been excreted by dogs, usually in the

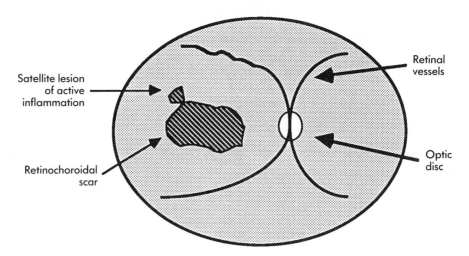

Fig. 6-8   Ocular toxoplasmosis may be manifested as an area of active retinal inflammation adjacent to an old scar.

soil in public playgrounds. Systemic infection usually goes unnoticed. Occasionally the syndrome of visceral larvae migrans results from the spread of the organism throughout the body. Typical features, which usually occur at 2 years of age, may include fever, cough, enlargement of the liver (hepatomegaly), and seizures. Ocular involvement is usually unilateral and occurs at an average age of 7 to 8 years. The eye findings may include the following.

Retinochoroidal granulomas. Retinochoroidal granulomas are whitish mass lesions involving the retina and choroid; they may be located in the posterior pole, midperiphery, or periphery. If the posterior pole is involved, vision will be diminished. If the granuloma is peripheral, the resulting vitreous traction can cause retinal detachment or the appearance of a dragged disc.

Chronic endophthalmitis. Chronic endophthalmitis is the most commonly seen condition, accounting for two thirds of all cases. A focal retinal granuloma is usually present associated with a localized retinal detachment secondary to serous exudation. The vitreous is filled with inflammatory cells (Fig. 6-9).

Tubular structure beneath the retina. A tubular structure appearing beneath the retina provides objective evidence of previous passage of the *Toxocara* worm through the eye. The diagnosis can be confirmed with the serum ELISA test, which yields a positive result in infected patients. However, seropositivity with no evidence of disease is common. In one study involving 333 kindergarten children, 30% were seropositive, but no one had evidence of ocular disease. Corticosteroids by mouth or by injection around the eye can be administered in the acute inflammatory phase. Laser photocoagulation can be used to kill a live worm outside of the macula if one suspects that it might turn and enter this vital area. Vitrectomy and retinal detachment repair may be necessary to improve vision. If the diagnosis of retinoblastoma cannot be ruled out by the characteristic calcifications detected with ultrasound, then an enucleation may be indicated.

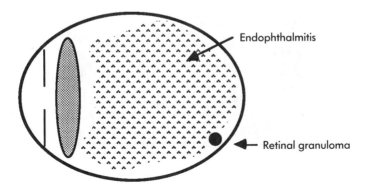

Fig. 6-9   Toxocara can result in a granuloma and associated chronic endophthalmitis.

CANDIDIASIS

Candidiasis is caused by the yeastlike fungus *Candida albicans*. Infection is more common in critically ill patients, patients with indwelling catheters, patients being treated with steroids or chemotherapeutic agents, or in IV drug abusers. Systemic infection may involve any organ. Multiple microabscesses may form in the bones, kidneys, intestinal tract, brain, and so on.

Ocular involvement is characterized by fluffy yellow-white lesions that usually start in the retina and spread into the vitreous. Diagnosis is made by this fundus picture associated with a history. The blood cultures may or may not yield positive results. Treatment is with antifungal agents, such as amphotericin, which can be administered by the intravenous periocular or intraocular routes.

SYPHILIS

This infection is caused by the spirochete *Treponema pallidum*. The disease may be congenital or acquired. The systemic manifestations of congenital syphilis include saddle-shaped nose, notching of the teeth (Hutchinson's sign), and deafness. The most common eye lesion is an interstitial keratitis (Fig. 6-10), which is caused by inflammation in the deep layers of the cornea. The inflammatory response usually occurs in the first or second decades of life and is thought to be an immune reaction against the treponemal organism located in the cornea. The other typical eye finding is a chorioretinitis, which gives a "salt and pepper" appearance to the fundus. The treatment of congenital

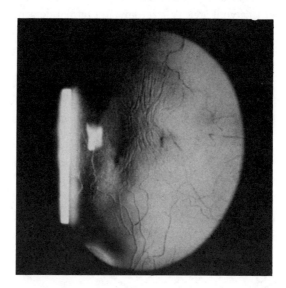

Fig. 6-10 The ingrowth of vessels in the deep layers of the cornea are manifestations of the interstitial keratitis of congenital syphilis. (From Stein H, Slatt B, and Stein R: Ophthalmic Terminology, ed 2, St Louis, The CV Mosby Co, 1987.)

syphilis involves large doses of antibiotics, such as penicillin. Topical steroids are used to control the corneal inflammation.

Acquired syphilis does not usually affect the eye. Inflammation involving the lids (blepharitis), iris (iritis), or iris and ciliary body (iridocyclitis) are the most common findings. Less common ocular manifestations include an interstitial keratitis and chorioretinitis.

The laboratory diagnosis of syphilis can be made by the Venereal Disease Research Laboratory (VDRL). The test usually yields a positive result in acute infections. The Fluorescent treponemal antibody Absorption test (FTA-ABS) will yield a positive result throughout the patient's lifetime.

7 Common neuroophthalmologic disorders

Neuroophthalmology is the branch of ophthalmology that deals with the nervous system associated with the eye. Making a neuroophthalmologic diagnosis is largely a procedure of localization—discerning the proper anatomic interruption in the sensory or motor pathways. For this reason, particular attention is drawn to the anatomy of the neuroophthalmic nerves and tracts and their surrounding structures (Fig. 7-1).

THE THIRD CRANIAL NERVE

The third cranial nerve is located at the level of the superior colliculi just beneath the grey substance. It has a V-shaped configuration in which the medial-longitudinal fasciculi form the lateral and central boundaries.

The third cranial nerve bundle, which arises from the ocular motor nuclei, passes ventrally through the brainstem and in so doing traverses the medial-longitudinal fasciculus, the red nucleus, and the substantia nigra to emerge in the interpeduncular fossa, that is, the angle formed by the peduncle and the pons. The third cranial nerve then travels through the subarachnoid space and enters the cavernous sinus just lateral to the posterior clinoid process. In the cavernous sinus, the third nerve travels with the other ocular motor nerves, namely the fourth and sixth cranial nerves, and emerges on the anterior part just lateral to the internal carotid artery. It penetrates the orbit through the superior orbital fissure and divides to the superior branch, which supplies the superior rectus muscle and the levator palpebral superioris muscle, and an inferior branch, which goes to the medial rectus muscle and inferior rectus muscle inferior oblique muscle. A small tributary goes to the ciliary ganglion.

CLINICAL FINDINGS
Total third-nerve palsy

Total paralysis of the third cranial nerve causes ptosis, loss of upgaze on the affected side, displacement of the eye downward or outward, and a fixed, dilated pupil that is unresponsive to light directed to the same side as well as to the opposite pupil.

Congenital third-nerve palsy rarely affects the entire nerve. It usually involves selected paresis of the levator and superior rectus muscles, either singly or together.

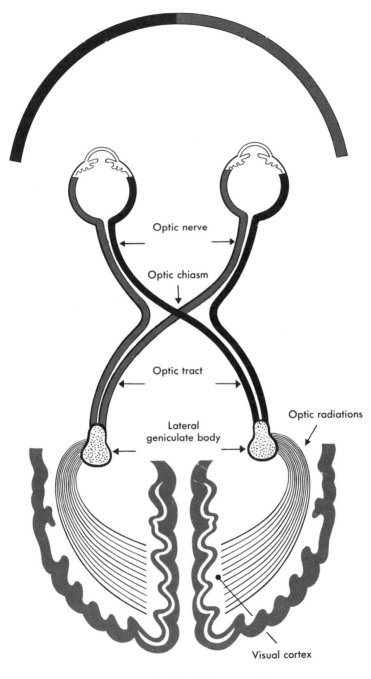

Optic nerve

Optic chiasm

Optic tract

Lateral geniculate body

Optic radiations

Visual cortex

Occipital lobe

7-1 Visual pathway. One-half the visual field from each eye is projected to one side of the brain. Thus visual impulses from the right visual field of each eye will be transmitted to the left occipital lobe.

Involvement of the third cranial nerve fibers as they pass over the red nucleus causes homolateral ocular motor paralysis with contralateral intension tremor (Benedikt's syndrome). Involvement of the third nerve at the level of the cerebral peduncle causes homolateral ocular motor paralysis and crossed hemiplegia (Weber's syndrome).

Cavernous sinus lesions are accompanied by disturbances in the other nerves to the orbit.

Cavernous sinus thrombosis

Cavernous sinus thrombosis produces a third-nerve palsy that may be diagnosed by the presence of marked exophthalmos, lid edema, and apparent sepsis.

Superior orbital fissure

Involvement of the superior orbital fissure causes unilateral paralysis of the third cranial nerve with a relatively small pupil, along with paralysis of the sixth and fourth cranial nerves. Frequently, the optic nerve is compressed as well. Tumors that can cause this condition include metastatic carcinomas, sphenoid ridge meningiomas, and nasopharyngeal tumors.

Diabetic ocular paralysis

Ocular paralysis related to diabetes comes on suddenly with involvement of usually a single ocular motor nerve. If the third cranial nerve is involved, the pupil is usually spared. The condition is frequently painful and results in diplopia. The paralysis usually lasts 6 to 8 weeks and resolves spontaneously. Sparing of the pupil is the indicator that the condition is largely vascular.

Aneurysm of the internal carotid artery

An aneurysm of the internal carotid artery can also produce a painful third-nerve ophthalmoplegia, but with involvement of the pupil. The pupil is fixed to light, both direct and consensual.

Migraine

Migraine can also produce a vascular type of third-nerve paralysis, with sparing of the pupil.

Thrombosis of the basilar artery

Basilar artery thrombosis can also yield a third-nerve paralysis. Any space-occupying lesion above the tentorium can cause impalement of the third nerve and ocular motor paralysis. At this position the pupillary fibers are most vulnerable, and mydriasis without a response to direct light may be the only sign.

Other tumors that may involve the third nerve include a pituitary adenoma, as it expands laterally, meningiomas of the sphenoid, and nasopharyngeal tumors.

Aberrant regeneration of the third cranial nerve can follow third-nerve paralysis. When the nerve fibers grow back, the alignment may not be correct. For instance, the new fibers that were destined for the inferior rectus may be misdirected and end up directed to the levator palpebral superioris, so that when a patient looks down, the lid retracts instead of the eye going down.

Aberrant regeneration of the third cranial nerve is a permanent condition. It can follow trauma, birth injuries, aneurysms, and tumors.

THE FOURTH CRANIAL NERVE OR THE TROCHLEAR NERVE

The fourth cranial nerve arises from the midbrain at the level of the midbrain at the position of the posterior colliculi—a paired group of motor cells just beneath the central gray substance. They are in virtual alignment with the third cranial nerve motor pool in the midbrain.

The fibers from the fourth cranial nerve have a dorsal exit and cross at the roof of the mesencephalon and emerge just behind the posterior colliculi. The fourth cranial nerves are the only motor nerves that rise dorsally and cross almost completely. When they emerge, they pass anteriorly and centrally above the superior aspect of the cerebral peduncles. They travel in the subarachnoid space and penetrate the cavernous sinus at the level of the posterior clinoid processes. In the cavernous sinus they travel closely with the other cranial nerves, namely the third and sixth, and pass through to the superior orbital fissure. The superior oblique muscle is innervated by the fourth cranial nerve.

Fourth-nerve paralysis

Fourth-nerve paralysis causes weakness of downward gaze and extortion of the eye. The fourth cranial nerve is an intorter and causes downward motion of the affected eye. In fourth-nerve paralysis, the patient tilts his head to the opposite shoulder to avoid seeing double. In congenital palsies of the fourth nerve, the head tilt may be so entrenched that it may cause torticollis.

Third- and fourth-nerve palsy

If the third nerve is involved, testing of the fourth nerve becomes difficult, because the eye cannot move medially and down. However, if the patient is directed to look up and down, the characteristic intortion of the eye on downward gaze will indicate an intact fourth cranial nerve.

The same conditions that involve the third nerve frequently involve the fourth nerve, especially with the superior orbital fissure involvement. There are, however, a few conditions that are rather specific to the fourth nerve. These include the following:
1. Fractures of the superior orbital rim, which causes displacement of the trochlea
2. Paget's disease, which also involves a mechanical disturbance of the trochlear process
3. Congenital fourth-nerve palsy

Clinical testing of the fourth nerve is performed by tilting the head, because palsies of the superior oblique and the superior rectus cause head tilting to the opposite shoulder. It is thus important to differentiate the involvement of these two muscles. The best criteria include the following:

1. Diplopia; with superior rectus palsies, the diplopia is maximal when the patient is looking up, whereas with fourth-nerve palsies it is greatest when the patient is looking down.
2. Head tilting is usually a feature of superior oblique palsy.
3. The eye is relatively elevated with a superior oblique palsy, whereas it is depressed with superior rectus palsy.
4. Bielschowsky's test.

Bielschowsky's head-tilt test

Bielschowsky's test differentiates between superior oblique palsy and contralateral superior rectus palsy. In certain long-standing cases, the patient is instructed to maintain fixation on a distant target and tilt his head to the side of the suspected superior oblique palsy while the behavior of the eye on that side is observed. If the eye is elevated, this is considered to be a positive response of the superior oblique muscle and is thought to have been the primary paralytic muscle. If there is no movement of the eye, the test result is considered to be negative, and no conclusion can be drawn as to which muscle was the original paralytic muscle.

THE SIXTH CRANIAL NERVE (THE ABDUCENS)

The sixth cranial nerve arises from paired motor cells from the floor of the fourth ventricle. The fibers of the facial nerve wrap around these nuclei to produce the facial colliculus. This sixth nerve motor pool also arises close to the pontine center for conjugate gaze and to the vestibular nuclei. Separating the two sixth-nerve nuclei are the medial-longitudinal fasiculi. The fibers of the sixth cranial nerve nuclei course ventrally without crossing to emerge from the brainstem at the posterior border of the pons. After emerging from the brain, they pass forward and laterally over the petreous tip of the temporal bone and alongside the dorsal sella to penetrate the cavernous sinus. They are the most lateral of the nerves that enter the cavernous sinus.

The sixth cranial nerve goes through the periorbital fissure and innervates the lateral rectus muscle.

Paralysis of the sixth cranial nerve

Paralysis of the sixth cranial nerve causes an inability to abduct the eye beyond the midline. Frequently the patient turns his head toward the side of the paralyzed muscle to avoid seeing double.

With fresh palsies of the lateral rectus muscle, the deviation is greater when the paralyzed eye is used for fixation. This is called *secondary deviation*. The deviation is actually smaller when the nonparalyzed eye is used for fixation. This is called *primary deviation*.

Paralysis of the sixth cranial nerve occurs with diabetes, lead poisoning, herpes zoster, and other previously mentioned conditions that involve the superior orbital fissure and the cavernous sinus.

Sixth cranial nerve paralysis is more likely to be accompanied by increased intracranial pressure. This is thought to result from the stretching of a nerve over the crest of the temporal bone.

Duane's syndrome. In Duane's syndrome there is a loss of abduction, retraction of the eye on attempted adduction, and with an occasional vertical displacement of the eye upon adduction.

Diabetes, meningitis, and skull fractures all can cause sixth nerve involvement.

Gradenigo's syndrome. Gradenigo's syndrome is characterized by a sixth-nerve palsy with pain on the side of the face. It is usually caused by a mastoid or middle ear infection.

Wernicke's encephalopathy. Wernicke's encephalopathy is frequently accompanied by a sixth-nerve palsy on one or both sides. This condition is fairly common in alcoholics who have a thiamine deficiency.

Brainstem lesions. Lesions involving the sixth and seventh nerves with varying degrees of nystagmus occur at the level of the sixth nerve motor pool.

Millard-Gubler syndrome results in a homolateral sixth-nerve paralysis and cross hemiplegia.

Diplopia. Diplopia is the most common symptom of a recently paralyzed muscle. Children who have misaligned eyes, either esotropia (inturning) or exotropia (outturning), learn to suppress the second image and do not suffer diplopia. However, any recently acquired extraocular muscle palsy invariably results in diplopia after the age of 5.

Basic rules for evaluating diplopia

1. Many patients will interpret blurred vision or a superimposed image as diplopia. With a true diplopia there are two images as a result of the misalignment of the two eyes not projecting to the same place in space. When one eye is covered, the second image or the alternate image will invariably disappear. If diplopia persists, it is more likely a pseudodiplopia and this may be related to cataracts, mucous deposits on the cornea, or simply result from blurred vision.

2. The patient should be asked if the two images are side by side or one on top of the other. If the images are separated horizontally, this restricts the possible affected muscles to the horizontal muscles namely the medial and lateral recti. If there is a vertical separation, this would indicate that the superior oblique, inferior oblique, and the superior and inferior rectus muscles are involved. If there is both a horizontal and vertical component, the horizontal component should be disregarded at first, since the paralysis of the vertical muscle may dissociate the eyes and permit underlying esophoria or exophoria to become manifest.

3. Bring the eyes to the position of extreme rotation, that is, abduction, adduction, or circumduction. For instance, if the maximum separation of the images is to the right, then that means that the left medial rectus muscle or right lateral rectus mus-

cle is at fault. Similarly, if there is a vertical separation of the image that is maximal when the patient looks down and to the left, the weaker muscle must be the left inferior rectus muscle or the right superior oblique.

4. Cover one image and see which one disappears. The distal image always belongs to the parietic muscle. For instance, if there is a right lateral rectus muscle paresis, then bringing the eye to the right would cause some limitation of abduction of the right eye. Therefore the image would be landing on the nasal side of the macula and be projected temporally to the most distal portion of the visual field. If the second distal image disappears by occluding the right eye, then the involved muscle would be the right lateral rectus muscle. If the diplopia fields were in a vertical direction and greatest with the patient looking down to the right and the image that was projected disappeared, then the parietic muscle would be the superior oblique muscle.

Another sign of diplopia is head turning that occurs with paresis of the lateral rotators. The head is invariably turned away from the paretic side. Head-tilting occurs with paresis of the superior oblique or superior rectus muscle. With palsies of the superior oblique or superior rectus, the tilting occurs toward the shoulder opposite the side of the parietic muscle.

Head-tilting is never as marked in superior rectus palsy as it is with superior oblique palsies.

Fixation also determines the degree of deviation. Fixation is usually determined by the visual acuity and refractive considerations. When the paralyzed eye is used for fixation, the deviation in the other eye is greater than when the normal eye is used for fixation.

If the magnitude of a deviation were the sole concern of the examiner, then an error would be made because the degree of deviation is greatest when the paralyzed muscle is used for fixation. In a lateral rectus palsy, the normal eye turns in.

LAG AND OCULAR MOVEMENT

A lag in ocular movement is most apparent with the horizontal muscles. In severe cases a lag in the motion of that muscle can be seen across the muscle field. In mild cases, there may be little visible lag.

At times it is easier to use a red-colored glass to identify the second image. This is placed over the patient's paralyzed eye to identify the second image. The measurement of the deviation in any position of gaze should be done with prisms to give a more accurate evaluation of the dimensions of deviation. It is also useful for follow-up studies when accurate numbers can be used for reference. It is important to establish for follow-up studies whether the paralytic eye or the normal eye was used for fixation. There should be consistency in this regard.

THE MUSCLES

The horizontal movements are controlled by the medial and lateral rectus eye muscles. These arise from the tendon of the zin, which is made up of extensions of periorbital

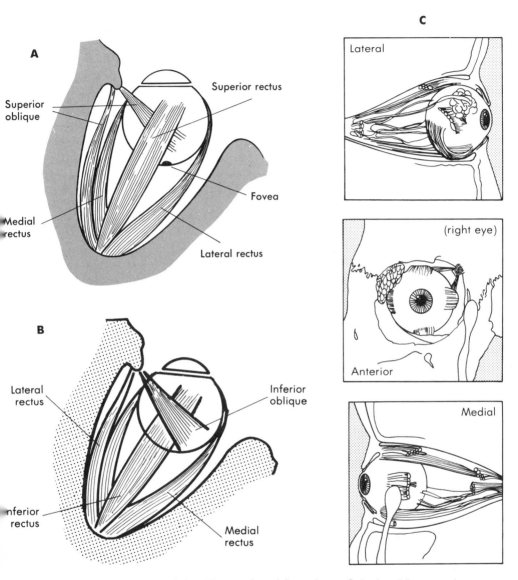

Fig. 7-2   A, Ocular muscles of the right eye viewed from above. Only the oblique muscles are inserted behind the center of rotation of the eye. All the recti muscles are inserted in front of the center of rotation of the eye near the limbus, where they are easily accessible for muscle surgery. **B,** Ocular muscles of the right eye viewed from below. **C,** The right eye viewed laterally, anteriorly, and medially.

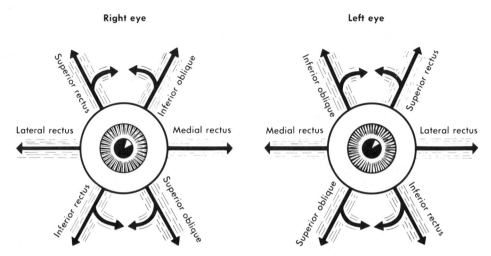

Fig. 7-3 Action of the extraocular muscles. The arrows reveal that the superior and inferior recti muscles function best as an elevator and a depressor, respectively, when the eye is abducted. The inferior and superior oblique muscles function best as an elevator and depressor, respectively, when the eye is adducted.

fascia. From the tendon of the zin are the superior and inferior rectus muscles. They fan out to insert to the globe approximately 5 to 8 mm from the limbus (Fig. 7-2). The superior oblique muscle extends from the apex of the orbit to the superomedial wall, where it is reflected by means of a tendon extension over a "pulley," the trochlea. It then passes underneath the superior rectus muscle and is inserted in the upper quadrant of the eye. The inferior oblique muscle has its origin in the lower portion of the anterior medial wall of the orbit directly below the trochlea. It passes below the inferior rectus muscle and is inserted on the lower quadrant of the eye.

The lateral rectus muscle rotates the eye outward or abducts the eye. The medial rectus muscle rotates the eye inward or adducts the eye. The superior and inferior rectus muscles are elevators and depressors of the eye when the eye is turned outward, whereas the inferior and superior obliques are elevators and depressors when the eye is turned inward (Fig. 7-3). The superior oblique muscle is a pure intortor and the inferior oblique muscle is a pure extortor. The superior oblique muscle also provides a secondary action to the adducting action of the eye, whereas the inferior rectus has a secondary action of abduction.

The movement of one eye from one position to another is called a *duction*. The movement of two eyes from the primary position to a secondary position is called *version*. Both eyes when moved to the right is called *dextroversion*; eyes to the left is *levoversion*; eyes up is called *sursumversion*; eyes downward is *dorsumversion* (Fig. 7-4 and Table 7-1).

Vergences is the term applied to simultaneous ocular movements in which the eyes

Table 7-1   Actions of extraocular muscles

Muscle	Primary action	Secondary action
Medial rectus	Turns eye inward toward nose, or adducts eye	None
Lateral rectus	Turns eye outward toward temples, or abducts eye	None
Superior rectus	Elevates eye	Intortion
		Adduction
Inferior rectus	Depresses eye	Extortion
		Adduction
Superior oblique	Intorts eye	Depression
		Abduction
Inferior oblique	Extorts eye	Elevation
		Abduction

are directed to an object in the midline in front of the face. This term is usually applied to convergence, in which the eyes rotate inward toward each other. Convergence is usually accompanied by narrowing or constricting of the pupils and accommodation. The triad of convergence, pupillary constriction, and accommodation is often called the *accommodative reflex*, although in the true sense they are merely the associated reactions. *Divergence* is the term used to indicate the eyes are moving outward simultaneously.

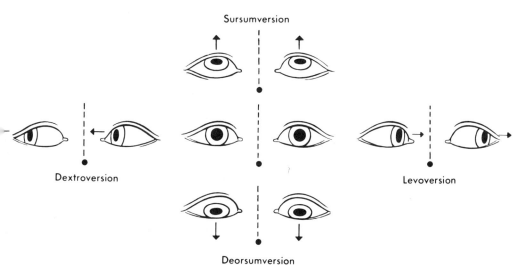

Sursumversion

Dextroversion

Levoversion

Deorsumversion

Fig. 7-4   Version movements of the eyes. These are movements formed by both eyes working together.

TYPES OF EYE MOVEMENT

Pursuit movements are following movements; they are slow, smooth, and gliding in nature, depending on the speed of the object that the eyes are tracking. Pursuit movements are controlled by centers in the occipital lobe of the brain.

Voluntary eye movements tend to be rapid, starting at high speeds and ending just as abruptly. Such movements occur with reading words or phrases that are quickly scanned, with an abrupt halt coming at the end of the section or line. These voluntary eye movements are controlled from the frontal lobe of the brain.

DISORDERS WITHIN THE EXTRAOCULAR MUSCLES
Thyroid—ophthalmoplegia

Ophthalmoplegia is a type of myopathy that can occur with hyperthyroidism or after treatment of hyperthyroidism with radioactive iodine. The characteristic clinical pathologic state is evident when a patient tends to look up—there is limitation of upward gaze.

The beta scan is quite useful for diagnostic purposes, because it reveals the thick and large extraocular muscles of thyroid disease.

In the congestive form of thyroid disease, the following signs may be present: retraction of the lids, retraction that is seen on downward gaze (the typical Graefe's sign), edema of the lids, congestion of the veins over the lateral recti muscles, exophthalmos, and loss of vision or pericentral scotomas.

Myasthenia gravis

Myasthenia gravis is characterized by diplopia in almost half of patients with the condition. Frequently a bilateral ptosis is the presenting symptom. The diplopia is variable and can mimic other conditions, such as the sixth-nerve palsy. Marked variability in diplopia is the signature of this disease. It is worse with fatigue and in the evening than in the morning. The diplopia can be horizontal or vertical, indicating different muscular involvements. This disorder appears to be an alteration in the acetylcholine cholinesterase mechanism, which may be deficient at the myoneural junction.

Hereditary ophthalmoplegia

Hereditary ophthalmoplegia is characterized by the gradual development of a restriction of ocular movement in all directions of gaze and ptosis. There is no pupillary involvement. The condition tends to run in families and occasionally is associated with retinitis pigmentosa.

The treatment of this disorder is strictly symptomatic. Ptosis surgery can frequently aid the drooping lids, which may cause loss of vision, whereas little can be done to alleviate the effects of the chronic loss of motility.

Pseudotumor of the orbit

Pseudotumor of the orbit is a disorder affecting the extraocular muscles and the orbit with chronic inflammatory cells. It is usually self-limiting and occurs primarily in young men. It is normally unilateral.

Supranuclear disturbances

Internuclear ophthalmoplegia is characterized by paralysis of the medial recti on attempted lateral gaze. It is caused by a lesion of the medial-longitudinal fasciculus. This tract extends from the third-nerve complex in the midbrain to the sixth-nerve complex in the pons. These tracts coordinate motor activities of the motor nerves of the eye with each other. Anterior lesions cause paresis of convergence, whereas posterior lesions of this tract cause weakness of the conjugate gaze and nystagmus. The nystagmus is asymmetric, being more marked in the abducted eye.

Bilateral internuclear ophthalmoplegia

Bilateral internuclear ophthalmoplegia causes loss of adduction or medial rectus paresis on both sides with attempted conjugated lateral gaze.

Unilateral types of this condition are usually the result of an occlusion of the small branch of the basal artery, whereas the bilateral form is invariably the result of multiple sclerosis.

Parinaud's syndrome

Parinaud's syndrome is characterized by paralysis of upward gaze, and to a lesser extent in downward gaze. The condition is found with lesions in the vicinity of the superior colliculi, primarily with tumors of the pineal gland. Associated disturbances include pupils that do not react to light but do react in near focusing.

Skew deviations

A skew deviation results from hypertropia that occurs with lesions in the general region of the posterior fossa. It is characterized by a maintained deviation of one eye above the other, which may be fixed or variable. The condition results from lesions of the brainstem or cerebellum. It occurs with bilateral internuclear ophthalmoplegia and is frequently found in the presence of cerebellar tumors or acoustic neuromas and compressive lesions (platybasia).

THE PUPIL

The pupil is made smaller (miotic) by the action of the sphincter muscle—a smooth muscle group situated in a circular manner within the iris stroma near the pupillary margin. This muscle is innervated by the parasympathetic nerves. The dilator muscle makes the pupil large (mydriasis) and is innervated by the sympathetic nerves to the eye. The dilator muscle is anterior to the pigment epithelium and lies near the periphery of the iris.

Mydriatic drugs dilate the pupil; these include epinephrine and cocaine. These are called *sympathomimetic* drugs. Drugs that paralyze the parasympathetic nerves include atropine and scopolimine. These cause mydriasis of the pupils. Drugs that excite the parasympathetic end organs include acetylcholine, pilocarpine, and mecholyl. These drugs cause miosis, or constriction, of the pupil.

The normal pupil should be round, regular, react to light and to accommodation and to near-point stimulation. The diameter of the pupil varies with the state of light adaptation. It enlarges in the dark and constricts in light. In a newborn the pupils are quite miotic, but at 3 weeks of age the pupils begin to enlarge. The relatively large size of the pupils is maintained during childhood until the third or fourth decade. By the fifth and sixth decade the pupil begins to get smaller again.

Pupillary tests

A direct light reaction consists of shining a light in the eye; the normal pupillary response is miosis or constriction.

A consensual light reaction results from shining a light in the opposite eye; it consists of miosis.

The near reaction is caused by a change in focus from a far to a near object and results in miosis.

Pupillary disturbances

An *amaurotic* pupil occurs in blind eyes and features the loss of direct light reaction with preservation of the consensual and near reactions. The consensual reaction from the blind eye to the normal eye is also absent. An amaurotic pupil occurs when blindness is caused by lesions in the retina or optic nerve.

Paralysis of the parasympathetic nerve supply

This results in a nonreactive pupil to light or near focusing. It occurs frequently with third nerve palsies as the parasympathetic nerve supply accompanies the third-nerve fibers. A fixed, dilated pupil is an important sign of subdural hematomas, temporal lobe tumors, and herniation of the brain contents against the tentorium. Pupillary fibers are subject to compression between the brainstem and the entrance into the cavernous sinus. With subdural hematomas, the mydriasis is invariably on the side of the subdural hematoma.

Paralysis of the sympathetic nerve supply

This results in relatively constricted pupil accompanied by ptosis of the upper lid and enophthalmus. Also, there may be loss of sweating on the affected side. This condition is called Horner's syndrome. Such a pupil still maintains a normal reaction to light and near fixation. This pupil is characterized by decreased sensitivity to mydriatic drugs such as cocaine or atropine, whereas the Horner's pupil shows a hypersensitivity to adrenaline. Adrenaline, one drop (1:1000 solution) in solution instilled three times over 10 minutes causes mydriasis and lid retraction on the affected side but not on the normal side. If the lesion causing Horner's syndrome is in the central nervous system, the pupil shows little sensitivity to adrenaline. Cocaine, one drop in four percent solution shows a diminished response on the side of the Horner's syndrome.

Peripheral Horner's syndrome can result from a variety of conditions including aneurysms, trauma, mediastinum tumors, aortic aneurysms and cervical lympanopathy.

With congenital Horner's syndrome, there is frequently an accompanying heterchromia so that the iris appears blue on the affected side whereas that on the normal side appears brown.

With combined sympathetic and parasympathetic lesions as occurs with cavernous sinus disturbances, the pupil is fixed and semidilated.

Pontine lesions

Pontine lesions create miosis and may be associated with disturbances of conjugate ocular movement. Pontine miosis may be caused by vascular accident, tumors, and multiple sclerosis.

Paratrigeminal syndrome

Paratrigeminal syndrome is characterized by pain in the face, tearing, and miosis. It may be caused by a vascular aneurysm.

Argyll Robertson pupil

In Argyll Robertson pupil, miotic reaction to light, either direct or consensual, is absent or sluggish. The miotic reaction is preserved with a near stimulus. In this condition pupils are frequently unequal in size; cocaine sensitivity is reduced. Argyll Robertson pupil is frequently found in syphilis of the central nervous system. Other less common causes are tumors of the pineal gland and encephalitis.

Adie's pupil

Adie's pupil consists of reduced constriction of the pupil with light or a near stimulation. The pupil recovers slowly with dilation in the dark. The condition often occurs unilaterally, but not always. It generally occurs in young women and is frequently associated with absent knee or ankle reflexes. The classic sign of Adie's pupil is that a fresh 2.5% solution of mecholyl instilled into the conjunctival sac will cause miosis and have no affect on the normal pupil.

NYSTAGMUS

Nystagmus is a disorder of eye movement characterized by involuntary, rhythmic oscillations.

Types of nystagmus

Pendular nystagmus is characterized by an oscillation that is approximately equal in rate in the two directions. Pendular nystagmus is converted to a jerk-type movement with a fast component to the side of the gaze. The cause of the nystagmus is poor vision in early infancy. Pendular nystagmus is found in the presence of the following conditions:

> Bilateral chorio-retinal lesions involving the macula in early infancy, such as toxoplasmosis
> Albinism with foveal aplasia

Aniridia with absence of the iris
Total color blindness (monochromatism)
Congenital cataracts
Congenital corneal scarring

Spasmeus nutans is a pendular nystagmus accompanied by head-nodding primarily in up and down gaze and occasionally torticollis. It may be unilateral and actually is the commonest cause of unilateral horizontal nystagmus in infancy. It appears in the first few months of life and lasts a matter of weeks or months.

Miner's nystagmus occurs in people who work in poorly lighted mines for long periods of time. This condition is rarely seen today. Hereditary nystagmus is a dominant sex-linked recessive trait. Voluntary nystagmus is a condition in which a person can cross his eyes to make extremely fine rapid horizontal oscillations.

In jerk nystagmus, the direction of the nystagmus is usually defined in terms of a fast component, since this is the most conspicuous one. Vestibular nystagmus may be horizontal, vertical, or rotary. If a nystagmus is maximal at the onset, it is probably caused by a peripheral lesion. Nystagmus from a vestibular nucleus in the brainstem remains static or increases. The coexistence of vertigo, skew deviation, and deafness is also indicated in a lesion of the brainstem or the eighth nerve.

Labyrinthitis (Meniere's disease) is accompanied by a rotary or horizontal nystagmus. Clinically there is a sharp onset of vertigo, nausea, and frequently tinnitus. There may be a skew deviation of the eyes with diplopia.

Conditions that frequently produce vestibular nystagmus include multiple sclerosis, encephalitis, Wernicke's disease, and some vascular disorders. The most frequent vascular disorder is a posterior and inferior vestibular thrombosis.

Alcoholism frequently causes nystagmus with other evidence of Wernicke's disease, sixth-nerve palsy, and gaze palsies.

Cerebellar tumors and abscesses also produce a vestibular type of nystagmus that varies with different positions of the head.

Other causes include intoxication with barbituates and analeptics.

Weakness of conjugate gaze. This type of nystagmus is frequently present to a slight degree in healthy people at the limits of mild gaze. It can be increased with alcohol intoxication. Otherwise, it is found in the recovery stage of palsies of conjugate gaze, and the nystagmus is invariably horizontal.

Congenital nystagmus. Congenital nystagmus is characterized by a turning of the head so that the eyes are in position of least nystagmus. The nystagmus is usually discovered in the first few months of life. It is invariably horizontal and usually causes some diminution of visual acuity, anywhere from 20/200 to 20/40.

Latent nystagmus. Latent nystagmus is a jerk type of nystagmus that is revealed by covering one eye or even flashing a bright light in one eye. Frequently, there is a jerk type of nystagmus and one eye turns inward. This type of nystagmus is important to recognize, because during visual acuity testing the uncovered eye will oscillate and the visual acuity will be diminished. The refraction of such patients can only be determined by obstructing the central vision with a card or some other obstructive device or by placing a +10 diopter lens over the untested eye.

THE SENSORY SYSTEM

The sensory system of the brain is quite orderly and begins with the nerve fiber layer of the retina, which is situated between the ganglion cells and the internal limiting membrane. This layer consists largely of the axons of the ganglion cells.

The axons of the ganglion cells travel horizontally toward the head of the optic nerve and the optic disc, and when they penetrate the lamina cribrosa of the optic nerve they become myelinated and form the optic nerve.

The temporal side of the optic nerve is occupied by those ganglion cells that radiate from the macula, which form the thinnest of the layers. There is less vasculature here, which explains why the normal optic disc when viewed ophthalmoscopically is invariably paler on the temporal side. The other fibers temporal to the disc sweep around the macular papullar bundle in an archlike form and penetrate the optic disc at the upper and lower poles, respectively. The nasal side of the disc is occupied by the fibers coming from the portion of the retina nasal to the optic disc.

Clinical correlates

1. The middle of the visual field corresponds to a line drawn through the macula, not through the optic disc.
2. The optic disc has no visual receptors and is the sight of the blind spot that can be detected on visual fields.
3. The retinal vessels emerge on the nasal side of the optic disc.
4. A full retinal vein pulsation of the surface of the disc invariably means that there is no increased intracranial pressure.
5. Because of the crush of fibers swooping around the macula to the upper and lower poles of the disc, these poles may normally be indistinct. The fuzzy margins should not be mistaken for edema.
6. Frequently, the fibers from the retina do not fill the entire optic nerve, and they leave the white scleral sievelike connective tissue membrane exposed. This is the lamina cribrosa, and it is a startling white color in contrast to the pinkish vascularized fibers of the tenth layer of the retina. This central white pit can vary in size and can have a sharp edge margin, a sloping edge margin, and can make the disc appear artificially pale. The ratio of exposed cup to the rest of the disc is used in glaucoma assessments and is called the *cup-disc ratio.*

THE ANATOMY OF THE ANTERIOR VISUAL SYSTEM

The optic nerve consists of myelinated nerve fibers that extend from the eyeball to the chiasm. It consists of (1) a portion within the sclera, (2) a portion that is in the orbit and has an S-like curve and is approximately 40 mm in length, (3) an intracanalicular part within the sphenoid bone, and (4) an intracranial portion that goes from the foramen of the sphenoid bone to form the chiasm.

Those fibers from the nasal portion of the retina, which is all the fibers nasal to the macula, cross over at the level of the chiasm, whereas the fibers temporal to the macula remain uncrossed.

Clinical correlates

1. Total compression of the chiasm, such as may occur with pituitary adenomas, will cause stretching and loss of function from the crossed intranasal fibers, which yield a bitemporal hemianopic defect, that is, a loss of the temporal side of each visual field. The optic nerve is surrounded by three vaginal sheaths called the *dura,* the *arachnoid,* and the *pia.* The dura is a tough, collagenous, compact connective tissue that is continuous with the periorbita and passes through the dura in the skull. The arachnoid consists of trabeculum, which contains the spinal fluid and forms a continuous passage into the intracranial space. The pia is the more delicate sheath consisting of fine collagenous fibers, elastic fibers, and endothelium, which invests the nerve and forms the scaffolding of the nerve. The blood supply of the optic nerve comes largely from the internal carotid system, which anastomoses with the external carotid system. From the internal carotid system is derived the ophthalmic artery, its major branches being the posterior ciliary arteries and the central retinal artery.

2. Total pallor of the disc is sometimes referred to as *primary optic atrophy.* Pallor of the disc may be associated with a central retinal artery occlusion, Tay Sach's disease in children (a lipid storage disease), and lead poisoning.

In children the most common lesion is a tumor of the orbit called a *glioma* of the optic nerve. The most common intracranial tumors in childhood that will cause a pale optic nerve are craniopharyngiomas, meningiomas, and ectopic pinealomas.

In adults the most common cause of pallor of the optic nerve is optic neuritis, probably secondary to multiple sclerosis. The most common ocular cause is glaucoma. Compressive lesions that can cause pallor include meningiomas, pituitary adenomas, cranial pharyngiomas, and metastases.

The clinical picture of pallor of the disc can be quite varied. After a central retinal artery occlusion, the entire optic disc is pale—almost chalk white—and the retinal arteries are attenuated. Immediately after a retrobulbar neuritis there may be absolutely no changes in the appearance or color of the optic nerve, but after 6 weeks or longer the optic nerve may become pale on the temporal side. With compressive lesions of the optic nerve, a field defect will often precede the change in color of the optic nerve.

PAPILLEDEMA

Papilledema is a mushroomlike elevation of the optic nerve head with a loss of detail in the optic disc margins. The elevation may protrude forward into the vitreous 4 to 5 diopters. This measurement is made by simply focusing with the ophthalmoscope on the head of the optic nerve and then focusing on the adjacent retina below it. The difference in the diopter value is a measure in diopters of the height in the optic nerve. To avoid employing one's accommodative power, the examiner should always use the highest plus lens in focusing.

Accompanying this swelling of the optic nerve are vascular changes that consist of distention of the retinal vein with hemorrhages and microinfarcts in the form of whitish exudates on the nerve fiber layer radiating around and about the disc. The hemorrhages and exudates are usually limited to within 1 to 2 disc diameters above the disc. If they extend into the macula, they assume a starlike configuration and appropriately are called the *macular star*.

Pseudopapilledema can be confusing when making a differential diagnosis. This is usually caused by buried amorphous matter called *drusen* in the substance of the optic nerve. However, it is rare to see the vascular changes, and the retinal veins are not distended and pulsate freely.

Optic atrophy occurs when resolution of papilledema takes place. The predominant findings are a pale disc with fuzzy disc margins created by the overgrowth of glial tissue. The retinal vein often shows a greyish sheathing that extends about a disc diameter from the disc itself.

Causes of papilledema

1. The most common cause of papilledema is increased intracranial pressure. This can result from tumors, such as large meningiomas and pinealomas of the midbrain. In children meningiomas must be suspected; cerebellar tumors and acoustic neuromas are other causes of papilledema.
2. Inflammatory disease of the optic nerve such as Guillain-Barré syndrome or infectious polyneuritis.
3. Subarachnoid hemorrhage and subdural hematomas.
4. Systemic disease; hypertension is the most common cause. Other causes include vitamin A intoxication and lead poisoning.
5. Pseuodtumor cerebri, a condition occurring in young to middle-aged adult, particularly women. It causes sixth-nerve palsy and headaches.

Other findings of the optic nerve

Other findings of the optic nerve include pits, which are isolated holes of the optic nerve. They are congenital and stationary. Also included are colobomas of the nerve head, usually situated in the lower corner of the disc, and staphylomas, which are outpouchings around the peripapillary region of the disc.

Retrobulbar neuritis

Retrobulbar neuritis is characterized by reduced visual acuity, pain on movement of the eye, a central scotoma, and a depressed pupillary reaction to direct light.

Approximately half of all patients with optic neuritis will eventually show signs of multiple sclerosis; 15% of patients with multiple sclerosis commence their disease with optic neuritis. Other conditions that may be present with the same symptoms are tumors of the orbit and aneurysms. A major differentiating feature is that with optic neuritis the visual acuity normally improves after 6 to 8 weeks, whereas with compressive lesions the visual acuity remains the same or deteriorates. Typically the optic disc is normal at the initial onset but after a period of 2 to 4 months the disc may develop characteristic temporal pallor.

Hereditary optic atrophy

Hereditary optic atrophy is also known as *Leber's optic atrophy*. This is usually a dominant type of transmission. Characteristically there is an abrupt onset, resulting in a change of visual acuity to 20/100 or 20/200. It appears normally in persons in their late teens or early twenties and is most often found in young men.

Behçet's disease

Behçet's disease is characterized by recurrent ulcers on the mouth, optic neuritis, and chronic uveitis.

Ischemic optic neuritis

Ischemic optic neuritis is often a feature of temporal arteritis. The onset is usually unilateral, although it can become bilateral. The diagnosis is confirmed by the presence of an elevated sedimentation rate or by a temporal artery biopsy that shows the characteristic giant cells in the temporal artery.

Tumors of the optic nerve

Tumors of the optic nerve are generally gliomas, which occur in the first decade of life and cause exophthalmos. It also causes unilateral loss of vision, optic atrophy, and occasionally paralysis of the extraocular muscles. These tumors do not metastasize; they are slow in growth potential. They may be associated with von Recklinghausen's disease and tuberous sclerosis (Bourneville's disease).

Meningiomas

Meningiomas arising from the sheaths of the optic nerve are uncommon, whereas those arising from the cranium itself are the most common. Meningiomas are more common in the age-group between 20 and 40 and are seen more often in women than in men.

The primary features of this condition are loss of vision and optic atrophy. Meningiomas within the orbit produce exophthalmos and various extraocular muscle palsies. Meningiomas can arise from the inner aspect of the sphenoid bone, from the tuberculum sella, or from the olfactory groove.

Differential diagnosis

Saccular aneurysms can involve the optic nerves. These arise generally from the internal carotid, the anterior cerebral and the anterior communicating artery. The unruptured aneurysm exerts compressive pressure on the optic nerve. They can result in central scotomas, blurred vision, and primary optic atrophy.

THE CHIASM

The anatomy of the area surrounding the chiasm is quite important because most common disruption in chiasmatic function results from compressive lesions surrounding it.

Just anterior to the chiasm is the lesser wing of the sphenoid; to the lateral side is the greater wing of the sphenoid. Posterior to it is the sella turcica. The lateral boundary of the chiasm is the internal carotid artery. The anterior cerebral arteries are dorsal to the optic nerves and superior to the chiasm. Tumor masses such as pituitary adenomas, meningiomas, and craniopharyngiomas can all compress the chiasm.

Classic findings of the chiasmal lesion

Bitemporal hemaniopia is the signature finding of a chiasmal lesion (Fig 7-5). Frequently, the major symptom is loss of visual acuity. Optic atrophy is a variable sign of chiasmic lesions. It may occur far after the onset of loss of vision; on the other hand, visual acuity may be remarkably preserved despite gross atrophy.

Headaches may occur, but these are usually associated with elevated intracranial pressure and occur with cranial pharyngiomas. Simple x-ray examination of the sella can be very helpful. These can reveal enlargement of the sella with intrasella tumors, calcification above the sella, which occurs with cranial pharyngiomas, and a thinning or thickening of the trabeculum sellas, as found with suprasellar meningiomas.

Summary

The posterior-superior portion of the chiasm contains the macular fibers.

The neuroophthalmic importance of the chiasm actually depends on the structures close to it. The chiasm is close to the pituitary gland, cavernous sinus, and the shenoid sinus; dorsal to it is the third ventricle.

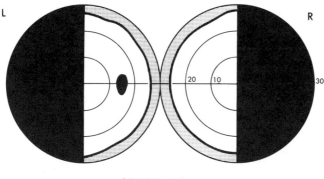

35/1000 White

Fig. 7-5 Bitemporal hemianopia.

Bitemporal hemaniopia is a characteristic field defect of all chiasmic lesions. Optic atrophy with chiasmal lesions is late and an unreliable sign. Other signs include ocular motor palsies and signs of endocrine disorders that are not related to the chiasm directly but rather to the pituitary itself.

Aneurysms, especially supraclinoid aneurysms derived from the internal carotid arteries, can produce blindness in one eye and temporal loss of vision in the other eye.

Trauma as occurs in traffic accidents can produce chiasmic disturbances largely through hemorrhages, ischemia, or thrombosis.

Pituitary adenomas, which occur in persons between 20 and 40 years of age, can cause gigantism or acromegaly; they can also cause chromophobic adenomas, which can lead to amenorrhea, impotence, loss of libido, fatigue, and hypoglycemia.

Cranial pharyngiomas arise from the vestiges of the hypophysial stock. They can produce signs of increased intracranial pressure and loss of vision. They also can create diabetes insipidus.

Meningiomas of the sphenoid or olfactory groove can involve the chiasm. They usually occur in persons between 30 and 50 years of age and are more frequently found in women. The tuberculum sella is actually the most common site of meningiomas. They are slowly progressive and benign.

The optic tract

The optic tract is the portion of the visual pathway that extends from the chiasm anteriorly to the geniculate bodies posteriorly. It forms an area that embraces the pituitary stock and the cerebral peduncles within its diverging arms.

The optic tracts are made up of fibers that are uncrossed on the temporal side of one eye and crossed from the nasal side of the other eye. The clinical features of tract lesions include the following:

• Hemianopia—a homonymous condition in which central acuity is normal
• Optic atrophy, which occurs weeks after the acute lesion
• Pupillary abnormalities, which consist of a larger pupil on the side opposite the lesion (Behr's sign).

The lateral geniculate body constitutes the end of the optic tract fibers. It in turn translates the visual impulses to the geniculocalcarian radiation to the calcarine cortex of the occipital lobe.

Geniculocalcarian radiation

The geniculocalcarian fibers, which emerge from the lateral geniculate body, fan out to embrace the lateral ventricle. The posterior medial portion of the tract, which has fibers from the upper retina, goes to the superior calcarine region of the occipital cortex. The fibers from the lower retina are deflected anteriorly to pass over the lateral ventricle of the temporal lobe before turning backward. The most anterior portion of this radiation is called *Meyer's loop.* These fibers terminate in the occipital cortex.

The macular fibers are represented in the posterior end of the calcarine fissure, whereas peripheral retinal fibers are found anteriorly. The connectors of the two halves of the brain are enveloped in the corpus callosum. The posterior portion of the visual cortex derives its blood supply from the posterior cerebral artery, whereas the anterior portion of the optic radiation gets its blood supply from the anterior choroidal artery and a portion of the middle cerebral artery.

Clinical findings

The most important finding of a lesion in this area is a homonymous hemianopia. There is no optic atrophy associated with these lesions. With lesions in the temporal lobe, the hemianopic defect begins in the upper quadrant at the visual field on the side opposite the lesion (Fig 7-6). With disturbances of the parietal lobe, they begin in the lower quadrant of the visual field on the side opposite the lesion.

As the lesions extend more posteriorly toward the occipital cortex, the hemianopic disturbances become more congruous (Fig 7-7); that is, they resemble one another so that one field defect can be superimposed on the other field defect on the other side.

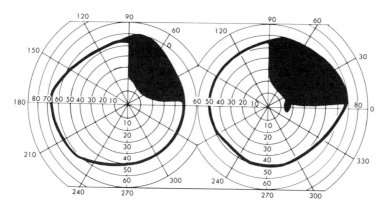

Fig. 7-6   Right incongruous homonymous superior quadranopia.

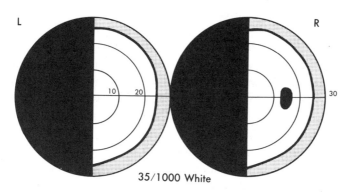

35/1000 White

Fig. 7-7   Left homonymous hemianopia.

The symptoms include a loss of vision; however, the patient may deny his blindness. The condition is called *Anton's syndrome.* There may be difficulty with reading. With a hemianopia on the right side, the patient is slow in reading. He cannot see words to the right of the point of fixation. A patient who has a left hemianopia can read across a line with ease but may have difficulty in skipping back to find the next line of print.

Signs and symptoms may be associated with a loss of function in the dominant hemisphere. The most common is the loss of the ability to read. This defect is called *alexia.* These patients have good recognition of visual symbols and excellent visual acuity to see what is being read. It may be associated with a loss of ability to write (*agraphia*), failure to recognize faces.

If a nondominant hemisphere is affected, there is a loss of spatial orientation. This occurs largely with disturbances in the parietal area. Patients with such a condition may lose their way home or even have difficulty dressing themselves. Neglect of the affected side is characteristic. This is seen with a patient when he attempts to draw a jar, clock, or face—one half of the diagram is usually left drawn. This is called *constructional apraxia.*

THE OCCIPITAL LOBE

The occipital lobes occupy the posterior portion of the cerebral hemisphere. They actually blend into the parietal and temporal lobes without any distinct anatomic landmarks. The calcarine fissure separates the upper and lower portions of the visual field. Central visual functions represented by the macula are interpreted at the occipital to represent of the posterior pole of the occipital lobe. The blood supply is largely derived from the posterior cerebral artery, which forms the terminal branches of the basal artery.

Clinical findings

The only reliable sign of occipital disease is a hemianopic defect (Fig. 7-8).

With bilateral lesions of the occipital lobe, the patient may be completely blind. Lesions of the occipital lobe never cause optic atrophy or a pupillary disorder.

Disturbances of the occipital lobe

1. Vascular lesions. Occlusion of one or both posterior cerebral arteries may occur through obstruction by an embolus or hemorrhage. Not only may there be signs of a homonymous hemianopia, but there can also be brainstem signs and symptoms as a result involvement of the basilar artery. These symptoms include diplopia, vertigo, dysphagia, ataxia, and palsies of conjugate gaze. Before the onset of these symptoms there may be transitory symptoms involving loss of momentary vision, anywhere from seconds to minutes in duration. Emboli arising from diseases of the heart, such as auricular fibrillation or disorders of the valves, may occlude the posterior cerebral arteries.

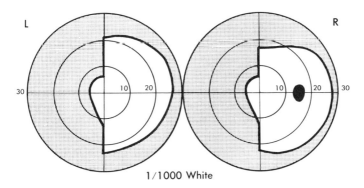

Fig. 7-8 Left congruous homonymous hemianopia.

2. Tumors of the occipital lobe include glioblastomas, metastatic tumors, and meningiomas.

3. Trauma. These can be caused by penetrating missiles and depressed bone fractures, which cause damage by direct and indirect injury. The most common injury is an inferior altitudinal hemianopia. Injuries to the posterior part of the occipital lobe cause central or pericentral scotomas. The most common cause of these injuries is an automobile collision.

4. Poisons that can affect the occipital cortex include carbon monoxide poisoning or digitalis, which causes a yellowness of the visual field.

5. Infantile cerebral blindness. Infantile blindness is difficult to detect, because the optic nerve tends to be pale at birth and the visual fixation responses during the first few weeks of life are similar to that of a seeing child. Eventually, at about 6 to 8 weeks of age, nystagmus may develop. This can be just a searching movement but soon the loss of visual fixation becomes apparent to the mother. Causes of blindness include cardiac arrest in infancy, Tay Sach's disease, cerebral agenesis, menigoencephalitis, and trauma, especially a subdural hematoma. The largest grouping of causes of intracranial blindness in infancy is hydrocephalus.

COMMON VISUAL DISORDERS
Cluster headaches

Cluster headaches are unilateral, occur predominantly in men, and are frequently accompanied by Horner's syndrome. They tend to recur in group attacks.

Migraine headaches

Migraine headaches are frequently preceded by an aura of scintillating or pulsating lights, or just a loss of vision centrally (Table 7-2). It can be unilateral or bilateral in its sensory effect and is followed by a headache lasting 1 or 2 hours. Migraines usually occur in families. Frequently they start in the first or second decades of life. However,

Table 7-2   Transient ischemic episodes (temporary loss of vision)

Duration	Cause	Findings	Tests
Seconds	Increased intracranial pressure	Papilledema	Fields enlarged
			Blind spot
	Hypertension	Attenuated retinal arterioles	Elevated blood pressure
1-3 minutes	Internal carotid artery occlusion	Emboli in retinal vessels	Doppler test
		Bruit in vessels of neck	
	Temporal arteritis	Ischemic optic neuritis	ESR elevated
10-20 minutes	Migraine	Normal eye examination	Field normal
Days to weeks	Multiple sclerosis	Feeble pupillary response to light	Central and paracentral scotoma

they can appear in an older age-group, and there is frequently just a visual aura without a headache.

Dyslexia

Dyslexia means difficulty with reading; it is a "wastebasket" term designated to include conditions from those that are strictly functional to those in which minimal brain damage has occurred. Such patients have excellent visual acuity but twist symbols, read words backward, such as *was* for *saw*, or omit portions of words so that a sentence becomes meaningless. Affected patients are frequently referred for an ophthalmic examination because the school suspects that some visual disturbance accounts for the child's poor reading skills.

Amblyopia

Amblyopia exanopsia is a reduction in vision occuring in an eye with strabismus. It occurs largely in children under 5 years of age in their attempt to avoid seeing double. The vision in the deviating eye is suppressed. Eventually the suppression becomes irreversible, and the loss of central vision is permanent. The loss of vision in a perfectly normal eye is called *amblyopia*. Amblyopia can also result from *anisometropia*, a condition in which the difference in the refractive error between the two eyes is greater than three diopters. Fusion of the two images may not be possible, so the brain suppresses the more out-of-focus image.

Examination of these children usually reveals completely normal eyes. There may be some pupillary defect in that the direct reaction to light may be slow or sluggish, and the Gunn's pupil sign may be present. That is constriction of the pupil may occur from exposure to light on the healthy side, whereas a feeble constriction followed by a dilation of the pupil may occur when the light is directed to the amblyopic side.

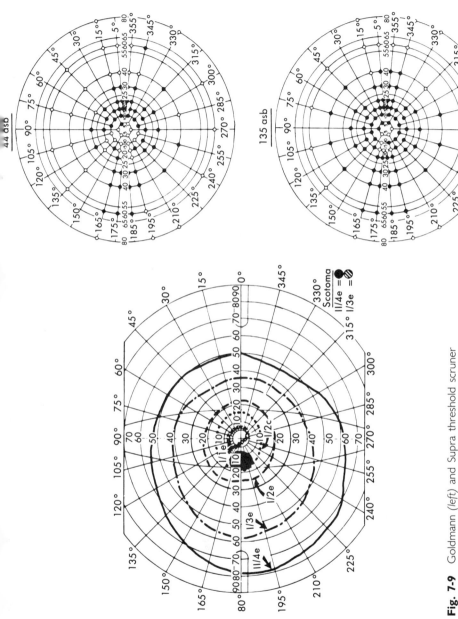

Fig. 7-9 Goldmann (*left*) and Supra threshold scruner (*right*) in a patient with nutritional amblyopia and a central scotoma.

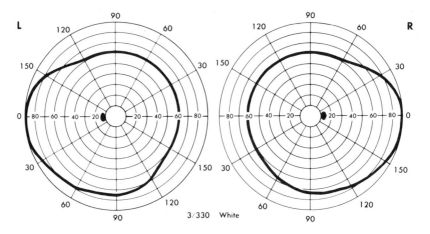

Fig. 7-10 Normal perimetric visual field.

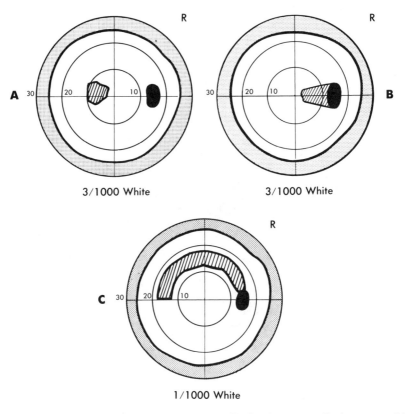

Fig. 7-11 Kinetic perimetry. **A,** Paracentral scotoma. **B,** Cecal scotoma. **C,** Arcuate, or Bjerrum, scotoma.

Static perimetry

Sensitivity of the retina can at any point be determined by presenting the patient with a test point of increasing light until the patient says that he can see the light. In static perimetry the field chart shows a profile of retinal sensitivity (Fig. 7-9). In that profile, the blind spot looks like a vertical tube (Fig. 7-10). The peak on a profile corresponds to an area of foveal fixation. Areas of loss of vision are mapped out as depressions, which can be shallow or deep below the normal range.

The charting of static perimetry must be done; eight meridians are usually obtained for charting, with a minimum of four at 90/180, 45/135 degrees. If defects are found, new areas can be explored.

Static perimetry is considered more accurate than kinetic perimetry, because charting retinal sensitivity is the more sensitive way of finding depressed areas of field defects.

Kinetic perimetry

Kinetic perimetry (Fig. 7-11) involves a moving target, whereas the background illumination is constant—the exact opposite of static perimetry. With kinetic perimetry the blind spot at 1 m is usually 5.5 degrees by 7.5 degrees high and is placed approximately 15 degrees temporal to the point of fixation. Because the field varies with the size of the target object and the visual acuity of the patient, both must be recorded.

With a 3 mm white target on the perimeter of 330 degrees, the average field of vision is 95 degrees outward and 75 degrees downward, 60 degrees inward and 60 degrees upward. With larger targets the lateral field can be pushed to about 110 degrees.

8 Management of ocular injuries and inflammatory eye conditions

NONTRAUMATIC RED EYE
Preseptal cellulitis

Preseptal cellulitis is characterized by erythema and swelling of the eyelids. The infection is confined to the anterior structures of the periorbita (Fig. 8-1).

Predisposing factors include a history of an upper respiratory tract infection, trauma to eyelids, or an external ocular infection. It must be differentiated from an orbital cellulitis, which can result in a permanent loss of vision. In a preseptal cellulitis the patient has normal vision, no proptosis, normal ocular motility, and no pain with eye movements. *Haemophilus influenzae* is the organism most commonly associated with this condition in children under 5 years of age, and *Staphylococcus aureus* and *Streptococcus* sp. in adults.

WORKUP
- Cultures are obtained from the nasopharynx, conjunctiva, and blood.
- The patient should be examined by an ophthalmologist to rule out orbital involvement.
- If the patient is unable to cooperate for the examination, or if there is any suspicion of orbital cellulitis, then a computed tomography (CT) scan should be ordered.

TREATMENT. *In mild to moderate cases the prescribed therapy for preseptal cellulitis is oral antibiotics:*
- In adults, cephalexin (Keflex) 250 mg q6h for 10 days.
- In children, cefaclor (Ceclor) 40 mg/kg/day (maximum 1 gm/day) q8h for 10 days.

In severe cases intravenous antibiotics are administered. For example:
- In adults, nafcillin 1.5 and penicillin 3 million units q4h.
- In children, ampicillin 200 mg/kg/day and chloramphenicol 11 mg/kg/day. If the organism proves sensitive to ampicillin, the chloramphenicol is discontinued.

Chalazion

Chalazion may be manifested initially as diffuse eyelid swelling which results from blockage of the duct of a meibomian gland (Fig. 8-2). Acutely, the obstruction may be secondary to infection by *Staphylococcus* sp. When the infection resolves, a painless nodule may remain that points to the skin or conjunctival side. Recurrent chalazia are often seen in association with blepharitis; appropriate treatment will decrease the incidence of this condition.

WORKUP. *There is effectively no workup for the treatment of this condition.*

TREATMENT

- Warm compresses can be applied for 10 minutes four times a day.
- Topical antibiotic such as Bleph-10 (sodium sulfacetamide) can be applied qid.
- If the condition does not resolve in 2 to 3 weeks and is of cosmetic concern to the patient, the affected area can be incised and drained with the patient under local anesthesia; infants and children usually require general anesthesia. The incision is usually made on the conjunctival side of the tarsal plate, which obviates a skin incision and resultant scar.

Acute dacryocystitis

Acute dacryocystitis is a blockage of the lacrimal duct that impedes the flow of tears through the lacrimal drainage system. Stasis occurs, which can result in a secondary bacterial infection and swelling and tenderness of the lacrimal sac (Fig. 8-3). The organism most commonly associated with this condition in children under 5 years of age is *Haemophilus influenzae* and in adults is *Staphylococcus aureus* (usually penicillinase-resistant).

WORKUP. *Pressure is applied to the lacrimal sac to express material through the puncta, and a conjunctival culture is prepared.*

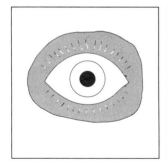 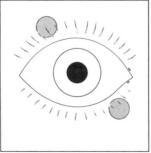 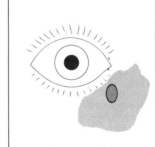

Fig. 8-1 Preseptal cellulitis is characterized by erythema and swelling of the eyelids.

Fig. 8-2 Chalazia are eyelid masses caused by obstruction of a meibomian gland.

Fig. 8-3 In acute dacryocystitis, blockage of the lacrimal duct causes swelling and tenderness of the lacrimal sac.

TREATMENT. *In mild to moderate cases oral antibiotics are prescribed:*
- In adults, Keflex 250 mg q6h for 10 days.
- In children, Ceclor 40 mg/kg (maximum 1 g/day) in divided doses every 8 hours for 10 days.

In severe cases intravenous antibiotics are administered as for preseptal cellulitis:
- Adults may receive nafcillin 1.5 g and penicillin 3 million units q4h.
- Children may receive ampicillin 200 mg/kg/day and chloramphenicol 11 mg/kg/day. If the organism is sensitive to ampicillin, the chloramphenicol is discontinued.
- When the infection resolves, a dacryocystorhinostomy is recommended to provide a drainage channel for the tears.

Blepharitis

Blepharitis is characterized by debris on the eyelashes, erythema of lid margins, and misdirection or loss of lashes (Fig. 8-4). It may be associated with conjunctivitis, keratitis, or neovascularization of the cornea. Blepharitis may be seborrheic, and/or secondary to *Staphylococcus* sp. Rarely, the lids may be infected by pediculosis.

TREATMENT OF STEPHYLOCOCCAL AND/OR SEBORRHEIC BLEPHARITIS
- Warm compress should be applied bid to the eyelids to remove scales, and the lid margins cleansed with dilute Johnson's Baby Shampoo applied with a Q-tip.
- Erythromycin ointment may also be applied to the eyelids at bedtime.
- Artificial tears are used if there is associated keratitis or dry eye, such as Tears Plus or Liquifilm Tears applied qid.
- If these measures fail to resolve the problem, then the patient should be referred to an ophthamologist.
- A short course of a topical steroid/antibiotic combination such as Blephamide may be useful, if there is significant inflammation.
- Tetracycline or doxycycline are useful in refractory cases.

TREATMENT OF PEDICULOSIS-ASSOCIATED BLEPHARITIS. *Pubic lice (pediculosis) involvement of the eyelids requires a distinct treatment:*
- A 20% fluorescein solution applied to lashes will cause the adult lice to fall off.
- Eggs must be removed manually.
- A 30% incidence of other venereal diseases exists, and this should be ruled out by appropriate testing.

Allergic conjunctivitis

Itching is the hallmark of allergic conjunctivitis. Other symptoms include tearing, redness, and chemosis (swelling of the conjunctiva), and the condition may be unilateral or bilateral (Fig. 8-5). The patient often has a history of allergies to dust, pollen, grass, cats, dogs, and so on.

WORKUP
- Conjunctival scraping is optional.
- Giemsa stain may show eosinophils.

Treatment

- Cold compresses, topical antihistamine and vasoconstrictors (such as Albalon-A qid) can be applied.
- If highly symptomatic, the patient should be referred to an ophthalmologist.
- A short course of a mild topical steroid (such as fluoromethodone [FML] qid) could be prescribed.

Adenoviral conjunctivitis

Adenoviral conjunctivitis is a highly contagious disease (for up to 10 days) character-ized by redness, tearing, and a variable degree of photophobia. Follicular hypertrophy of the conjunctiva, which is difficult to detect in the absence of a slit lamp, microscopi-cally represents focal collections of lymphocytes. Keratitis may be absent or limited to superficial punctate keratitis or subepithelial infiltrates (Fig. 8-6). The enlarged preau-ricular lymph nodes are helpful in the diagnosis as they are never seen in bacterial con-junctivitis except with the gonococcal organism.

Workup. *Cultures are unnecessary, since diagnosis is based on clinical evaluation.*

Treatment

- No specific antiviral therapy is available.
- Cold compresses can be applied for patient comfort.
- Artificial tears (such as Tears Plus qid) or astringents (such as Albalon-A qid) can be used.
- Prophylactic precautions should be observed by the patient's family members and friends.
- Children should stay away from school for 7 to 10 days.
- If the examiner is uncertain of the diagnosis, it should be assumed that the cause is bacterial, and the condition treated with a topical antibiotic.

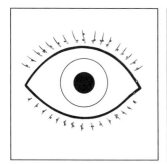 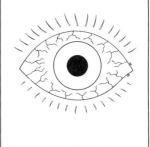 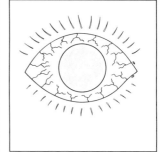

Fig. 8-4 Blepharitis is charac-terized by debris on lashes, er-ythema of lid margins, and mis-direction or loss of lashes.

Fig. 8-5 Allergic conjunctivitis is characterized by itching, red-ness, and chemosis.

Fig. 8-6 In adenoviral con-junctivitis the keratitis may be absent or limited to superficial punctate keratitis and/or subep-ithelial infiltrates.

Bacterial conjunctivitis

The symptoms of bacterial conjunctivitis are redness and purulent discharge (Fig. 8-7). There is no preauricular node enlargement except in cases of gonococcal conjunctivitis. This condition is less common than viral conjunctivitis.

WORKUP. *In severe cases or those involving a neonate, a Gram stain and culture can be prepared.*

TREATMENT

- Broad-spectrum antibiotics are prescribed, such as Sodium Sulamyd qid.
- In children under 5 years of age infection may be by *Haemophilus influenzae*, and Choroptic or Bleph-10 can be used as treatment.
- In cases of gonococcal conjunctivitis, the patient is admitted to hospital, and may be treated with intravenous antibiotics and topical application of bacitracin every half-hour.

Chlamydia

This is a venereal disease that is usually seen in young sexually active adults. The ocular symptoms of chlamydial infection include redness and mucoid discharge, with or without photophobia. The preauricular lymph nodes may be enlarged (Fig. 8-8). Follicular hypertrophy of the conjunctiva is characteristically seen by slit lamp examination, and later in the disease course a superior micropannus of the cornea may develop. This condition is refractory to topical eye medications, and unlike adenoviral conjunctivitis that usually resolves in less than 1 month, it may become chronic if not treated.

WORKUP

- The patient should be referred to an ophthalmologist.
- Clinical diagnosis is made based on the signs and chronicity.
- A Giemsa stain, culture, and fluorescent antibody stain can be performed, but false negatives may occur.

TREATMENT. *The standard treatment for this problem is oral:*

- Tetracycline 250 mg qid for 1 month.
- The patient's sexual partner must be similarly treated for the same duration.

Herpes simplex

Primary herpes simplex

The first exposure to herpes simplex virus in 90% of cases results in subclinical, usually mild disease. Resistance increases with age, so that primary infection is exceedingly rare in early adult life. Characteristically, the young child is infected by salivary contamination from an adult who has labial herpes. The incubation period is 3 to 9 days. The clinical features of herpes simplex are both ocular and nonocular.

Ocular disease. Characteristics are vesicular eruption (especially lower lid and medial canthus), conjunctivitis, regional lymphadenopathy, and occasional corneal epithelial disease (Fig. 8-9). Symptoms are frequently unilateral.

Nonocular disease. The following forms of the disease may be present:

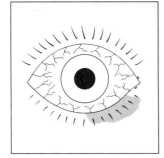
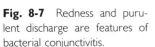

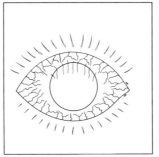

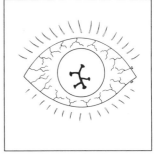

Fig. 8-7 Redness and purulent discharge are features of bacterial conjunctivitis.

Fig. 8-8 Chlamydial infection is characterized by redness, mucoid discharge, follicular hypertrophy, and superior micropannus as seen by slitlamp examination.

Fig. 8-9 Dendrite is the characteristic feature of herpes simplex keratitis.

- Gingivostomatitis—The symptoms are fever, malaise, cervical lymphadenopathy, and sore throat.
- Pharyngitis—In college students, a primary attack of herpes simplex virus frequently results in a pharyngitis with vesicles on the tonsils.
- Cutaneous disease—Generally, type I occurs above the waist and type II below the waist. This disease may be seen in wrestlers, rugby players, and as a herpetic whitlow in dentists.
- Genital infection—Type II of the infection is more common than type I and is characterized by balanitis in males and cervicitis/vulvovaginitis in females. Patients may exhibit fever, myalgia, extensive vesicular lesions, and inguinaland pelvic lymphadenopathy.

Recurrent herpes simplex

The virus develops a "symbiosis" with man, and trigger mechanisms such as trauma, fever, sunlight, emotional stress, steroids, and menses provoke viral shedding, and immunological functions may be overcome. The trigeminal ganglion is a reservoir for the type I disease. The virus has a 50% recurrence rate over 5 years, and the recurring condition may be highly localized on the lips, nose, chin, eyes (lids, conjunctiva, corneal epithelium, corneal stroma, uvea), and genitals.

WORKUP. *Since this is a clinical diagnosis, cultures are usually unnecessary.*

TREATMENT. *The various forms of herpes simplex require specific treatment:*

- *Blepharitis* may occur without conjunctival or corneal disease. If it is recurrent, this is consistent with herpes simplex; herpes zoster does not recur. If there is involvement of the skin but not the lid, no topical antiviral treatment is necessary. If the lid margin is involved, then prophylactic antivirals (such as Viroptic 5 times per day) are applied to the conjunctiva.

- *Conjunctivitis* may occur without lid or corneal disease and the patient may have an enlarged preauricular lymph node. Ophthalmic referral is recommended and an antiviral (such as Viroptic 9 times per day) may be applied.
- *Keratitis* occurs in the following forms:

Punctate keratitis is characterized by raised clusters of opaque epithelial cells, as evidenced with fluorescein stain. Referral to an ophthalmologist is recommended. If diagnosis is unequivocal, a topical antiviral (such as Viroptic 9 times per day) may be applied. In the case of an equivocal diagnosis, treatment should be deferred and the patient followed closely.

Dendritic keratitis is recognized by desquamation in the center of plaques of swollen epithelial cells. The typical linear branching ulcer (stains with fluorescein) has overhanging margins of swollen opaque cells, which are laden with virus (stains with rose bengal). Ophthalmic referral is recommended and an antiviral (such as Viroptic 9 times per day) should be applied.

Geographic keratitis results from progression of dendritic keratitis; a geographic epithelial defect (stain with fluorescein) is lined by heaped-up opaque cells (stain with rose bengal) and may be associated with steroid use in dendritic keratitis. Ophthalmic referral is recommended and an antiviral (such as Viroptic 9 times per day) should be applied.

Stromal keratitis is an immunologic disease characterized by corneal stromal infiltrates and/or edema. Corneal inflammation that may be associated with iritis and keratic precipitates results from antibodies directed at viral antigens. Ophthalmic referral is recommended. If the epithelium is intact, a topical steroid, such as Pred Forte 5 times per day and an antiviral cover (such as Viroptic 5 times per day) may be applied. If the stromal keratitis is associated with an epithelial disease, an antiviral (such as Viroptic 9 times per day) should be applied until the epithelium heals (approximately 14 days), after which a topical steroid can be added.

Herpes zoster

Herpes zoster tends to occur in children under 14 and in adults over 40 years of age. Its incidence is five times greater in those over 80 years of age than in adults between 20 and 40. A 50% incidence of AIDS has been found in male patients between the ages of 20 and 40 in New York City. The development of herpes zoster may be the first manifestation of AIDS.

The varicella virus which causes chickenpox can lie dormant in the sensory ganglia and later reactivate as shingles or herpes zoster. Causes of reactivation are unknown but may be related to aging, immune compromise (for example, AIDS, lymphoproliferative diseases, systemic steroids), and trauma to the involved ganglion. Although chickenpox is contagious, it should not cause herpes zoster; however, children can develop chickenpox after contact with herpes zoster patients. Once the virus is reactivated, it may be contained (zoster sine herpete), or spread to the brain, skin, eye, or enter the bloodstream. The virus has a predilection for dermatomes T3-L3, but the most common site is the trigeminal nerve. Cutaneous lesions of herpes zoster are histopathologically identical to varicella but have a greater inflammatory reaction, which can cause scarring. The dermatome pattern of herpes zoster may occur in three sites supplied by branches of the trigeminal nerve:

- The ophthalmic nerve distribution (V1) where it occurs 20 times more frequently than at the V2 or V3 sites. Frontal involvement is the most common, including the upper lid, forehead, and superior conjunctiva, which are supplied by supraorbital and supratrochlear branches (Fig. 8-10). Alternatively, it may spread to the lacrimal and nasociliary area, which supplies the cornea, iris, ciliary body, and the tip of the nose.
- The maxillary nerve distribution (V2).
- The mandibular nerve distribution (V3).

The virus may affect none, any, or all of these branches. Involvement of the nasociliary nerve often leads to infection of the eye. Hutchinson's rule (1860s) states that ocular involvement is frequent, if the side of the tip of the nose is involved.

Clinically, herpes zoster is characterized by a prodrome, skin disease, and ocular complications. The patients may experience pain, burning, itching, hyperesthesia in the dermatome area, followed by erythema, macules, papules, and vesicles that become confluent and may form deeply pitted scars (dermis affected by necrotic process). Ocular complications include lid scarring and exposure, muscle palsies, conjunctivitis, episcleritis, scleritis, keratitis, uveitis, and retinitis.

WORKUP. *Systemic evaluation for underlying malignancy is not indicated, since the yield is low.*

TREATMENT

- Compresses can be applied to the affected areas of the skin.
- Medication for pain relief can be given.
- Antivirals may be prescribed: acyclovir 600 mg given orally 5 times per day for 10 days may prevent serious ocular disease and may accelerate resolution of skin lesions. It is more effective if it is started within 72 hours of the onset of the disease and it has no effect on preventing postherpetic neuralgia. Topical antiviral therapy is ineffective treatment for the eye.
- Systemic steroids (such as prednisone) for 2 to 3 weeks may be prescribed for patients over 60 years of age, since this is the age group most susceptible to postherpetic neuralgia. However, steroids may cause disseminated herpes zoster and therefore should not be given in immunodeficient patients.
- The patient should be referred to an ophthalmologist to rule out ocular involvement.
- Topical steroids (such as Pred Forte qid) will improve comfort and decrease the chance of corneal scarring.
- Cycloplegic agents (such as Cyclogyl, 2%, bid) will relieve ciliary spasm in corneal and anterior chamber inflammation making the patient more comfortable and dilating the pupil to prevent posterior synechiae (iris-lens adhesions).

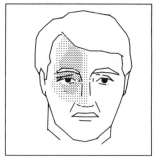

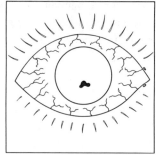

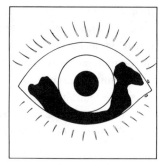

Fig. 8-10 Herpes zoster ophthalmicus is characterized by vesicular skin eruptions in the distribution of any of the branches of the trigeminal nerve.

Fig. 8-11 Recurrent corneal erosions stain with fluorescein.

Fig. 8-12 A ruptured vessel with blood accumulation in the subjunctival space is diagnosed as a subconjunctival hemorrhage.

Recurrent corneal erosions

Patients with recurrent corneal erosions experience pain, photophobia, and redness, but have no acute history of trauma. Corneal erosion, which stains with fluorescein (Fig. 8-11), is due to the lack of strong corneal epithelial attachments. The erosion frequently occurs on awakening, since the corneal epithelium becomes more edematous during eyelid closure and more susceptible to focal sloughing. Predisposing factors for this condition may be an old traumatic injury (such as fingernail, tree branch, paper), corneal dystrophy, and bullous keratopathy (that is, corneal edema).

WORKUP. *No workup is required.*

TREATMENT

- Antibiotic ointment or drops (such as Sodium Sulamyd) and a cycloplegic agent (such as Cyclogyl, 1%) should be prescribed.
- A pressure patch should be applied.
- Ophthalmic referral is recommended.
- Hypertonic drops and/or ointment, such as sodium chloride 5% drops during the day and ointment at bedtime to be used over a period of weeks to months to dehydrate the epithelium and decrease the risk of erosions.
- Anterior stromal puncture can be performed if the patient continues to develop erosions in the same location. A 25-gauge needle can be used to make multiple punctures into the anterior stroma in the area of the erosion. This allows for the development of stronger adhesions and decreases the risk of erosions. However, the technique is contraindicated in erosions that occur close to the pupillary axis.

Subconjunctival hemorrhage

A ruptured vessel with blood accumulation in the subconjunctival space describes a subjunctival hemorrhage (Fig. 8-12). It is often accompanied by a history of coughing, vomiting or straining. The patient may be taking coumadin or aspirin.

WORKUP

- If the patient's history is negative for Valsalva maneuvers, a blood pressure reading should be taken.
- The patient on coumadin should undergo tests to ensure that the rate of blood clotting is in the desired range.
- In the case of recurrent subconjunctival hemorrhage, a complete blood count should be taken to rule out a blood dyscrasia.

TREATMENT. *Reassuring the patient is all that is necessary, since the hemorrhage will resolve spontaneously.*

Phylectenule

A phylectenule is a small pinkish-white nodule in the center of a hyperemic area of conjunctiva (Fig. 8-13). Although it is seen most frequently near the limbus, it may occur anywhere on the bulbar conjunctiva. Less commonly, it involves the cornea where it is associated with vascular ingrowth. The patient's history should be used to rule out the possibility of any foreign body. Phylectenules may be caused by a hypersensitivity reaction to an antigenic stimulus such as *Staphylococcus aureus* or the tubercle bacillus.

WORKUP

- The patient should be referred to an ophthalmologist.
- A tuberculin skin test and chest x-ray evaluation are recommended if the patient is in a high-risk group.

TREATMENT

- A topical steroid (such as Pred Forte qid) may be prescribed.
- Any associated staphylococcal blepharitis should be treated.

Episcleritis

Episcleritis is characterized by a salmon-pink hue of the superficial layer of the eye, with involvement of the conjunctiva and episclera (Fig. 8-14). At least one third of the lesions are tender to touch. Simple episcleritis may be sectorial in 70% or generalized in 30% of the patients. In nodular episcleritis, unlike in nodular scleritis, the nodules that form are movable with a Q-tip.

WORKUP. *Ophthalmic referral is recommended.*

TREATMENT. A topical steroid (such as FML or Pred Forte qid) will cause resolution of the inflammation.

Scleritis

Scleritis is frequently bilateral and, characteristically, associated with pain. The ocular surface has a purplish hue with involvement of the deep episcleral vessels (Fig. 8-15).

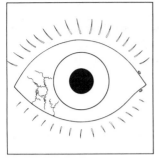 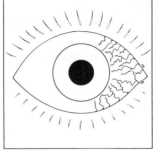 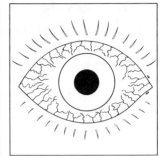

Fig. 8-13 Phylectenules are small, pinkish-white nodules surrounded by conjunctival hyperemia that occur most frequently near the limbus.

Fig. 8-14 Sectoral episcleritis is characterized by a salmon-pink color of the conjunctival and episcleral tissues.

Fig. 8-15 A purplish hue and injection of conjunctival and deep episcleral vessels are signs of scleritis.

Systemic diseases, such as collagen vascular, ulcerative colitis, Crohn's disease, and sarcoidosis, are present in 50% of patients. Eight-year mortality is 30%, with death usually resulting from a vascular disease. Scleritis may be classified as simple (in its most benign form), nodular (the nodule is immobile when pushed with a Q-tip), or necrotizing (the majority of these patients have rheumatoid arthritis).

WORKUP
- Ophthalmic referral is recommended.
- The patient should be evaluated for an underlying systemic disease.

TREATMENT
- A topical steroid (such as Pred Forte) may be prescribed to reduce the inflammation.
- A systemic nonsteroidal anti-inflammatory medication is recommended (such as Indocid 25 mg orally tid).

Corneal ulcers

Patients with corneal ulcers may experience redness, pain, photophobia, and tearing. The cornea will have a whitish infiltrate with an overlying epithelial defect that will stain with fluorescein (Fig. 8-16). Patients most at risk are those who wear contact lenses, those with blepharitis and dry eyes, or those who have experienced corneal trauma. The most common causes are bacterial infections, for example, by *Pseudomonas*, *Staphylococcus aureus*, or *Streptococcus pneumoniae*.

WORKUP
- Ophthalmic referral is recommended.
- The cornea should be scraped for Gram stain and culture.

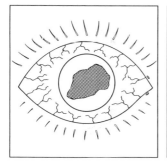 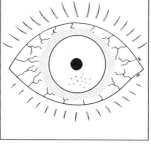

Fig. 8-16 Corneal ulcers— the epithelial defect that overlies the whitish corneal infiltrate stains with fluorescein.

Fig. 8-17 In iritis ciliary flush is prominent, the pupil is constricted, and slitlamp examination reveals keratic precipitates.

TREATMENT. *Topical fortified antibiotics, for example, tobramycin (15 mg/mL) and cefazolin (50 mg/mL) can be applied.*

Iritis

Iritis is characterized by redness, photophobia, tearing, and decreased vision. A ciliary flush is prominent and the pupil is constricted as a result of the inflammation (Fig. 8-17). Slit lamp examination shows an anterior chamber reaction manifested by inflammatory cells and flare (protein leakage), and keratic precipitates. Testing with fluorescein stain should be done to rule out a corneal abrasion and herpes simplex dendrite.

WORKUP

- Ophthalmic referral is recommended.
- If condition is persistent or recurrent, underlying systemic disorders (for example, ankylosing spondylitis, sarcoidosis) should be ruled out.

TREATMENT. *A topical steroid (such as Pred Forte q1-2h) and a cycloplegic agent (such as Cyclogyl 1% or homatropine 5% q6h) should be prescribed.*

Acute angle-closure glaucoma

Acute angle-closure glaucoma is characterized by redness, severe pain, photophobia, and decreased vision (Fig. 8-18); the patient may also experience nausea and vomiting. Elevated intraocular pressure, corneal edema, and a nonreactive mid-dilated pupil may also be present. This tends to occur more frequently in the hyperopic (far-sighted) eye because of a relatively narrow anterior chamber.

WORKUP

- Tonometry should be performed to confirm diagnosis.
- Ophthalmic referral is recommended.

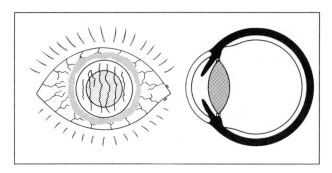

Fig. 8-18 Acute angle-closure glaucoma is manifested by elevated intraocular pressure, associated with redness, ciliary injection, corneal edema, a nonreactive middilated pupil, and a relatively narrow anterior chamber angle.

TREATMENT
- Effective medications include: pilocarpine 2% q5min ×4, then q1h; Betagan drops q12h; isosorbide 1-2 g/kg orally ×1; Diamox 250 mg orally q6h or 500 mg IV; mannitol 20% 1-2 g/kg IV.
- Laser iridotomy can be performed in the affected eye and a prophylactic iridotomy in the contralateral eye.

TRAUMATIC RED EYE
Corneal abrasions

The patient with a corneal abrasion has a history of trauma caused, for example, by a tree branch, fingernail, or contact lens. The patient will complain of pain, photophobia, redness, and blurred vision.

WORKUP. *The diagnosis is confirmed by demonstrating an epithelial defect with fluorescein dye (Fig. 8-19).*

TREATMENT
- Antibiotic drop or ointment (such as Bleph-10) should be instilled along with a cycloplegic agent (such as Cyclogyl 1% or homatropine 5%).
- A pressure patch should be applied.
- Analgesic medication may make the patient more comfortable.
- Patient follow-up is recommended on a daily basis to determine epithelial healing and ensure the absence of an infection.

NOTE: Contact lens–related abrasions should not be patched, because a subclinical infection may be present. Instead, these abrasions should be treated with antibiotic drops active against *Pseudomonas* (such as tobramycin q2h).

Contact lens

Contact lens wearers may develop a red eye as a result of a variety of pathophysiologic causes: mechanical, hypoxic, immunologic, chemical toxicity, and infection. The most

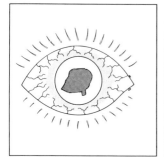

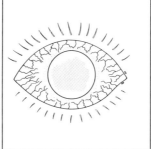

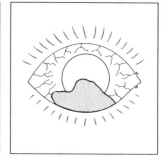

Fig. 8-19 Corneal abrasion is characterized by an epithelial defect (which stains with fluorescein) and ciliary injection.

Fig. 8-20 Ultraviolet keratitis is characterized by a superficial punctate keratitis, which stains with fluorescein associated with ciliary injection and blepharospasm.

Fig. 8-21 Depending on the type and severity, signs of chemical injury may include conjunctivitis, superficial punctate keratitis, epithelial defects of the cornea and conjunctiva, blanching of blood vessels, and necrosis of tissues.

important concern is the possibility of the development of an infected ulcer, which can lead to corneal scarring and a permanent decrease in vision.

WORKUP. *Refer to Appendix E for the differential diagnosis of red eye in contact lens wearers.*

TREATMENT

- All patients with a red eye should remove their contact lenses.
- Referral to an ophthalmologist is necessary to determine the cause of red eye.

Ultraviolet keratitis

Ultraviolet keratitis is usually bilateral and is characterized by redness, photophobia, tearing, and blepharospasm (Fig. 8-20). Usually the patient has been welding or using a sunlamp without proper eye protection. Typically, the symptoms appear 6 to 10 hours after exposure.

WORKUP. *Fluorescein staining will reveal the presence of superficial punctate keratitis.*

TREATMENT

- An antibiotic drop or ointment (such as Bleph-10) should be instilled along with a cycloplegic agent (such as Cyclogyl 1%).
- The more severely affected eye should be patched and the patient instructed to apply a patch to the less affected eye at home.
- A pain medication can be prescribed.
- Follow-up is recommended to ensure epithelial healing.

Chemical injuries

Alkali injuries are often more severe than acid injuries, because acids tend to coagulate tissue and inhibit further penetration into the cornea. Clinical findings of chemical injury vary with severity of the injury: a mild injury is characterized by conjunctivitis, superficial punctate keratitis, and an epithelial defect of the cornea and conjunctiva; a severe injury exhibits blanching of limbal blood vessels and opacification of the cornea (Fig. 8-21).

Alkali agents

- Ammonia—Commonly found in household ammonia (7% cleaning agent), fertilizer, and refrigerant (strongest concentration is 29%). Penetration of the eye occurs in less than a minute, which makes the injury difficult to treat by irrigation.
- Lye (sodium hydroxide)—Commonly found in drain cleaners (for example, Draino), it ranks second to ammonia in severity of injury induced.
- Hydroxides—Common forms are potassium hydroxide (found in caustic potash) and magnesium hydroxide (found in sparklers and flares). The chemical burns are similar to those caused by sodium hydroxide.
- Lime ($CaOH_2$ = calcium hydroxide)—This is one of the most common substances involved in ocular burns and is found in plaster, cement, mortar, and whitewash. However, because it reacts with the epithelial cell membrane to form calcium soaps which precipitate, it penetrates the eye poorly.

Acid agents

- Sulfuric acid (H_2SO_4)—Commonly found in batteries and industrial chemicals, injuries are often caused by battery explosions with resultant lacerations, contusions, and foreign bodies. When H_2SO_4 comes into contact with the water in the corneal tissue, heat is released charring the tissue and causing severe injury.
- Sulfur dioxide (SO_2)—Commonly found combined with oils in fruit and vegetable preservatives, bleach, and refrigerant. It forms sulfurous acid (H_2SO_3) when it combines with water in corneal tissue. Injury is caused by the H_2SO_3 rather than the freezing effect of SO_2; it denatures proteins, inactivates numerous enzymes, and penetrates tissue well because of its high lipid and water solubility.
- Hydrofluoric acid (HF)—Commonly used for etching and polishing glass or silicone, frosted glass, refined uranium and beryllium, alkylation of high octane gasoline, production of elemental fluoride, inorganic fluorides, and organic fluorocarbons. Much of the damage to the eye is caused by the fluoride ion.
- Other acids—These include chromic acid, hydrochloric acid, nitric acid and acetic acid.

WORKUP. *Since this emergency situation requires immediate treatment, no workup is recommended.*

TREATMENT. *The emergency physician should initiate the following procedures:*

- The eye should be irrigated with a nontoxic liquid (water, ionic solutions, buffered solutions), but acidic solutions are not recommended because they are too risky. An IV drip for at least 30 minutes is recommended with the eyelids retracted. The pH can be checked using litmus paper, although this is optional.

- Any particulate matter should be removed from the fornices. A moistened Q-tip can be used to remove chemical matter.
- A cycloplegic agent (such as Cyclogyl or homatropine) will prevent posterior synechiae and alleviates ciliary spasm.
- An antibiotic ointment can be applied, along with a pressure patch.

The ophthalmologist may initiate the following treatment:

- The patient should be followed closely to ensure the healing of the epithelium.
- The intraocular pressure should be lowered if it is elevated (for example, prescribe Betagan and/or Diamox).
- Topical steroids may be used to decrease inflammation but should be limited to no more than 2 weeks in the case of a persistent epithelial defect. Prolonged steroid use in the presence of an epithelial defect can cause the cornea to melt.
- Bandage contact lenses may be used, if the epithelium is not healed by patching.
- If the cornea heals with scarring and vascularization, the prognosis for restoring vision using a corneal transplant is poor because of the high incidence of graft rejection and failure.

Corneal foreign bodies

A corneal foreign body may be present in the patient exhibiting redness, foreign-body sensation, photophobia, and a history of trauma (Fig. 8-22).

WORKUP. *None is required.*

TREATMENT

- A topical anesthetic should be instilled and the foreign body removed with a needle (for example, 22-gauge) or a burr drill. If the foreign body cannot be seen, the upper lid should be everted to examine the lid margin and the palpebral conjunctival surface.
- A cycloplegic agent (such as Cyclogyl 1%) should be instilled, along with an antibiotic drop or ointment (such as Bleph-10).
- A pressure patch should be applied.
- Follow-up is recommended to determine epithelial healing, and to ensure the absence of infection or residual rust.

Intraocular foreign bodies

A small, foreign body traveling at a high speed can penetrate the eye without the patient's awareness. The symptoms are highly variable, depending on the site of penetration and intraocular structures affected. All foreign bodies made of iron should be removed, since they can cause significant intraocular damage (siderosis bulbi). However, glass, aluminum, gold, and silver are inert and usually cause little or no chronic intraocular damage (Fig. 8-23).

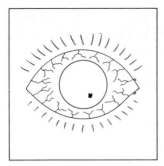 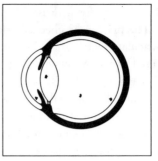

Fig. 8-22 Redness, foreign-body sensation, and photophobia occur in the presence of a corneal foreign body.

Fig. 8-23 Intraocular foreign bodies can be found in a variety of sites: in the anterior chamber, lens, vitreous, or retina.

WORKUP
- An x-ray examination (Waters' view and lateral) should be ordered if an intraocular foreign body is suspected.
- Ophthalmic referral is recommended.
- If the foreign body cannot be visualized on examination, a CT scan should be ordered to determine whether the foreign body is intraocular or extraocular.

TREATMENT. *To extract an intraocular foreign body, magnetic extraction or vitrectomy with foreign body instrumentation is usually indicated. Most foreign bodies outside of the eye in the orbit can usually be left without adverse sequelae.*

Blowout fracture

A blow to the periorbital structures can cause a fracture of the orbital floor and result in periorbital ecchymosis, infraorbital nerve anesthesia, and limitation of up-gaze. There are two theories as to the mechanism of a blowout fracture: (1) That a blow to the orbit causes a sudden increase in intraorbital pressure, which results in the fracture, and (2) a blow to the inferior orbital rim, which results in a buckling of the orbital floor.

WORKUP
- An x-ray examination (Waters' view and lateral) and a CT scan (anteroposterior and coronal views of orbits) should be taken.
- Ophthalmic referral is recommended.
- The eye should be checked for any associated intraocular damage (for example, hyphema, scleral rupture, traumatic cataract, macular edema, choroidal rupture, retinal tears, or retinal detachment).

TREATMENT
- Patients should try to refrain from nose-blowing and coughing.

- Systemic antibiotics should be prescribed (such as Keflex 250 mg orally qid for 10 days).
- Surgical repair of the orbital fracture depends on the CT scan findings and/or clinical signs during the subsequent 1 to 2 weeks.
- Surgery is indicated in cases of soft tissue entrapment associated with diplopia, enophthalmos greater than 2 mm, and fractures involving more than half the orbital floor.

Hyphema

Hyphema is usually caused by trauma from a blunt object and is characterized by decreased vision, ciliary injection, and a view of the fundus which is hazy because of the presence of blood (Fig. 8-24). Children often have an unreliable history, and it is important to rule out any intraocular foreign body. A tear in the ciliary body or iris usually occurs in the area of the angle. The incidence of rebleeds is 20% to 25%, usually between the third and fifth day.

WORKUP. *No workup is recommended.*

TREATMENT

- Ophthalmic referral is recommended.
- A protective eye shield should be applied.
- Hospital admittance should include bed rest with bathroom privileges.
- A cycloplegic agent and antiglaucoma medication should be prescribed.
- Aminocaproic acid (Amicar) reduces the incidence of secondary hemorrhage and may be taken orally by the patient.
- Patients should be told that they are at an increased risk for the development of glaucoma secondary to damage to the angle, as well as for retinal detachment. Therefore patients should be followed on a regular basis for the rest of their lives.

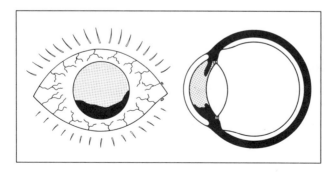

Fig. 8-24 Usually the result of blunt trauma, hyphema (or blood in the anterior chamber) is characterized by decreased vision, ciliary injection, and a hazy view of the fundus because of the presence of blood.

Blunt trauma injury

Hyphema, cataract, iridodialysis, scleral rupture, traumatic mydriasis, choroidal rupture, retinal tears and/or retinal detachment may be present in blunt trauma injuries.
WORKUP. *No workup is required.*
TREATMENT
  • Ophthalmic referral is recommended.
  • A protective eye shield should be applied.
  • Cataracts, scleral ruptures, retinal tears, and/or retinal detachments should be surgically managed.
  • Any associated hyphema should be treated as previously described.

Lacerations

WORKUP. *No workup is required.*
TREATMENT
  • Ophthalmic referral is recommended.
  • A protective eye shield should be applied.
The following are the treatment options, depending on the affected sites:
  Lid—If the lid margin is involved, a suturing technique is critical to prevent notching.
  Conjunctiva—If an isolated injury, repair is usually unnecessary.
  Sclera—Always suspect a puncture or laceration when the conjunctiva is involved; scleral laceration requires sutures and treatment with intravenous antibiotics to prevent endophthalmitis.
  Cornea—Full-thickness lacerations require sutures, and puncture wounds that leak can be glued with tissue adhesives.
  Lens—Cataract extraction is indicated for this injury.
  Vitreous—A vitrectomy should be performed.

DECREASED VISION IN WHITE EYE

The emergency physician should be able to make the diagnosis of a sudden decrease in vision. Early treatment of central retinal artery occlusion and ischemic neuropathy secondary to giant cell arteritis can be sight-saving.

Vein occlusion

The presence of scattered superficial retinal hemorrhages may indicate a central retinal vein occlusion (CRVO) or a branch retinal vein occlusion (BRVO) (Fig. 8-25). In CRVO the hemorrhages are located primarily at the posterior pole but may be seen throughout the fundus; in BRVO the hemorrhages are located in the distribution of the occluded vein.
WORKUP
  • Ophthalmic referral is recommended.
  • The intraocular pressure in both eyes should be taken, since patients with vein occlusions have a higher incidence of glaucoma.

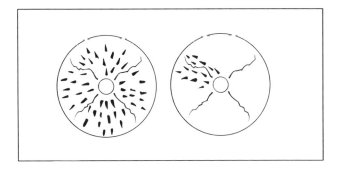

Fig. 8-25 Scattered superficial retinal hemorrhages are indicative of *left:* central retinal vein occlusion or *right:* branch retinal vein occlusion.

- Fluorescein angiography may be performed to determine the extent of retinal ischemia and/or macular edema.

TREATMENT
- In CRVO, panretinal laser photocoagulation is indicated, if the retina shows significant ischemic change. This technique prevents the neovascularization of the anterior chamber angle which can lead to glaucoma.
- In BRVO, focal laser photocoagulation may improve visual acuity and may be indicated for chronic macular edema. If neovascularization of the retina develops, then focal laser photocoagulation may resolve the neovascular tufts and prevent a vitreous hemorrhage.

Artery occlusion

Both central retinal artery occlusions (CRAO) and branch retinal artery occulusions (BRAO) are characterized by ischemic whitening of the retina. In CRAO the fovea appears as a cherry-red spot, since the choroidal vasculature is easily visible through this relatively thinned retinal area (Fig. 8-26). Central visual acuity may rarely be normal in CRAO, if the blood supply from the choroidal vasculature to the fovea is maintained by a small retinal artery (cilioretinal artery). Most occlusions are caused by emboli that may be seen on the disc in CRAO or in an artery in BRAO.

WORKUP
- The patient's history should be taken to determine whether cerebral transient ischemic attacks have occurred.
- The carotid arteries and the heart should be evaluated to determine the source of the emboli.

TREATMENT
- Less than 4 hours by history is a true emergency.
- The patient should be given an ocular massage, along with Betagan drops, Diamox 500 mg orally, and mannitol 20% 200 mL IV.
- Ophthalmic referral is recommended.

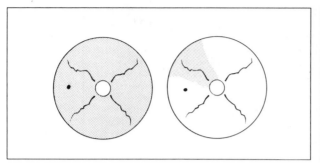
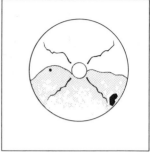

Fig. 8-26 Ischemic whitening of the retina is indicative of *left:* a central retinal artery occlusion or *right:* a branch retinal artery occlusion.

Fig. 8-27 In retinal detachment the retina appears white when elevated. If the macula is detached, the central vision will be diminished.

Retinal detachment

When a retinal tear develops, fluid may accumulate beneath the retina, creating a retinal detachment. A visual field deficit is present and the retina appears white when elevated (Fig. 8-27). There is an increased risk of retinal detachment in patients with myopia, aphakia, pseudophakia, or previous ocular trauma.

WORKUP. *No workup is required.*

TREATMENT

- Ophthalmic referral is recommended.
- Surgical correction is required.
- If the patient's vision is diminished (that is, the macula is detached), there appears to be no difference in final visual acuity whether the surgery is performed immediately or after 2 or 3 days.

Maculopathy

A sudden decrease in vision, often associated with *metamorphosia* (wavy vision), suggests a macular problem. The macula may be affected by edema, hemorrhage, and/or exudates. Differential diagnosis includes diabetes mellitus, macular degeneration, histoplasmosis, and central serous retinopathy.

WORKUP

- Ophthalmic referral is recommended.
- Fluorescein angiography may be performed to determine the source of macular leakage.

TREATMENT

- If leaking vessels and/or microaneurysms are identified in diabetic patients, laser photocoagulation can be performed.

- In the case of choroidal neovascularization in macular degeneration or histoplasmosis, laser photocoagulation can be applied if the vessels are not directly beneath the fovea.
- In central serous retinopathy, a fluorescein angiogram will often identify a focal leakage point of the retinal pigment epithelium which causes an accumulation of fluid beneath the retina. The majority of cases resolve spontaneously. However, the course can be shortened by using a laser to seal the defect in the pigment epithelium.

Vitreous hemorrhage

Vitreous hemorrhage is characterized by a hazy view of the fundus. The most common causes are posterior vitreous detachment, proliferative diabetic retinopathy, vein occlusion with neovascularization of the retina, retinal tear without detachment, retinal detachment, macroaneurysm of the retina, and trauma.

WORKUP
- Ophthalmic referral is recommended.
- A B-scan ultrasound should be taken to rule out associated retinal detachment and/or mass lesions such as a malignant melanoma.

TREATMENT
- The majority of hemorrhages will resolve spontaneously in a few weeks to months.
- Vitrectomy may be indicated in nonclearing vitreous hemorrhages. It may also be combined with laser photocoagulation if there is an associated retinal tear or neovascularization, or a scleral buckle if there is a retinal detachment.

Optic neuritis

Optic neuritis is usually seen in patients between 20 and 50 years of age, who complain of a decrease in vision and pain with eye movement. Patients usually have decreased color vision. The optic disc is swollen or it may appear normal in retrobulbar optic neuritis (Fig. 8-28). Of these patients, 40% will develop multiple sclerosis.

WORKUP
- Ophthalmic referral is recommended.
- The visual field should be checked and a follow-up test performed to determine the course of visual loss.
- If the initial visual field is atypical or if vision does not improve over 6 weeks, a CT scan should be taken to rule out a compressive lesion.

TREATMENT
- No specific ocular therapy is generally indicated.
- Controlled studies of systemic steroids have failed to demonstrate any difference in long-term outcome between treated and untreated groups. However, steroids have been shown to shorten the duration of the acute attack in some patients. Therefore patients with visual loss in both eyes may benefit from steroidal therapy, such as prednisone 80 mg/day tapered over 2 to 3 weeks.

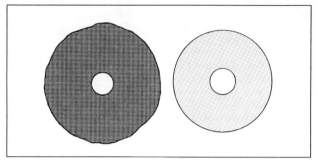 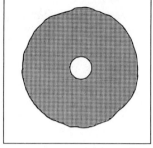

Fig. 8-28 Optic neuritis is characterized by *left:* a swollen optic disc and indistinct disc margins; or *right:* a normal appearing disc in retrobulbar optic neuritis.

Fig. 8-29 Ischemic optic neuropathy is accompanied by a pale swelling of the optic disc and indistinct disc margins.

Ischemic optic neuropathy

Ischemic optic neuropathy is usually seen in patients over 50 years of age and is characterized by a sudden decrease in vision and a swollen optic disc (Fig. 8-29). The disease process is idiopathic in the majority of cases. Occasionally the condition is secondary to giant cell arteritis (GCA). This is an inflammatory condition of medium to large arteries with a predilection for extradural cranial arteries including the ophthalmic vessels. The symptoms and signs of GCA are headache, jaw claudication, and temporal artery tenderness, but it is important to note that patients with GCA may exhibit only visual symptoms.

WORKUP
- The erythrocyte sedimentation rate (ESR) should be obtained to rule out GCA. In this condition the ESR is usually elevated.
- Temporal artery biopsy is the definitive test to confirm the diagnosis.

TREATMENT
- No specific treatment exists for idiopathic ischemic optic neuropathy.
- Ophthalmic referral is recommended.
- If GCA is present, systemic steroids should be started immediately to protect the patient from bilateral visual loss.
- Steroids are usually tapered and maintained for a minimum of 9 to 12 months.

DIPLOPIA
Third nerve palsy

The third nerve innervates four eye muscles: the superior rectus, medial rectus, inferior rectus, and inferior oblique. It carries the parasympathetic fibers to the sphincter of the iris and innervates the levator muscle of the upper lid.

In third nerve palsy there may be diplopia, ptosis, and/or a dilated pupil. The eye is deviated out and down. The etiology of this condition is as follows: aneurysm 20%, vascular disease (diabetes, hypertension, atherosclerosis) 20%, tumors 15%, trauma 15%, and miscellaneous and undetermined 30%.

WORKUP

- If the pupil is fixed and dilated, other causes should be ruled out (for example, Adie's pupil, or contamination with a dilating drop).
- If the pupillary dilatation is secondary to third nerve palsy, this constitutes a medical emergency and neurosurgical referral is required. Cerebral angiography and CT scan should be ordered to rule out intracranial aneurysm or neoplasm. If the pupil is not involved, diabetes, hypertension, collagen vascular disease, and giant cell arteritis (if the patient is more than 55 years of age) should be ruled out.

TREATMENT

- Ophthalmic referral is recommended.
- The eye can be patched to alleviate diplopia.
- The majority of third nerve palsies not involving the pupil resolve within 6 months.
- If muscle weakness persists for more than 12 months, surgery can be performed to improve *cosmesis* (cosmetic appearance).

Fourth nerve palsy

The fourth nerve supplies the superior oblique muscle which moves the eye downward and inward. The palsy causes elevation of the eye with resultant vertical diplopia and involves a torsional component making images appear tilted. Congenital fourth nerve palsies may initially be asymptomatic, and a head tilt may be the only symptoms. As image fusion ability diminishes over time, diplopia results. Acquired fourth nerve palsies are usually caused by head trauma.

WORKUP

- If the fourth nerve palsy is isolated, it is not necessary to test for any underlying systemic diseases.

TREATMENT

- Ophthalmic referral is recommended.
- Prismatic correction in eyeglasses or surgical intervention may be indicated, depending on the severity and the duration of the palsy.

Sixth nerve palsy

The sixth nerve innervates the lateral rectus muscle, which moves the eye out. A palsy is characterized by horizontal diplopia (images side-by-side), most prominent in the field of gaze of the underactive lateral rectus muscle. The patient may be partially or completely unable to move the eye laterally.

WORKUP

- Obtain a patient history; children often have a history of a recent viral illness or immunization.
- In adults, diabetes, hypertension, collagen vascular disease, and GCA (if over the age of 55) should be ruled out.
- If sixth nerve palsy is not isolated (that is, associated with other nerve palsies) or if the patient has papilledema, then a CT scan is indicated to rule out a neoplastic process.

TREATMENT

- Ophthalmic referral is recommended.
- Isolated sixth nerve palsies usually resolve spontaneously within six months.
- An eye patch can be placed over the affected eye, or if the patient wears eyeglasses, tape can be placed over the lateral portion of the lens.
- If muscle weakness persists for more than 12 months, surgery can be performed to align the eyes in primary gaze.

9 Clinical atlas

The following color atlas will give you the opportunity to see a full array of common ophthalmological diseases. Unlike diseases that occur within the human body, many disorders of the eye can be detected by direct observation. An old saying, "a picture is worth a thousand words," has been one of the main thrusts of this text. It was our aim to attach a common atlas of eye disorders in color so that one could readily identify common diseases and disorders. This chapter serves that purpose.

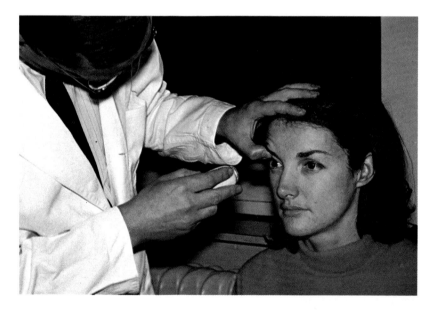

Fig. 9-1 Examination of the external portion of the eye is performed by using a hand penlight and holding up the upper lids as shown. On external examination, note whether the eye is white or red. Are the pupils reacting normally? Does the cornea look lustrous and clear or is there some scar tissue or haze present? Examine the eye for proptosis. Examine the lids as to whether they fall within the normal alignment. The upper lid should cross approximately one millimeter of the colored iris, while the lower lid lines up against the lower margin of the iris.

All illustrations in this chapter from Bedford MA: *Color atlas of ophthalmological diagnosis*. London, England, 1986, Wolfe Publishing Ltd.

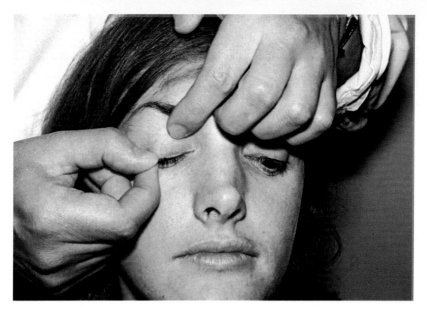

Fig. 9-2 Evert the upper lid to detect foreign bodies and papullar or follicular reaction of the conjunctiva. The best method is to stand behind the patient as shown. On everting the upper lid, always have the patient look down to relax the levator muscle. Then pull the lid outward by grasping the lashes and everting the lid over the index finger of the opposite hand. Alternatively, one can use a Q-tip on the upper border of the tarsal plate while everting the lid.

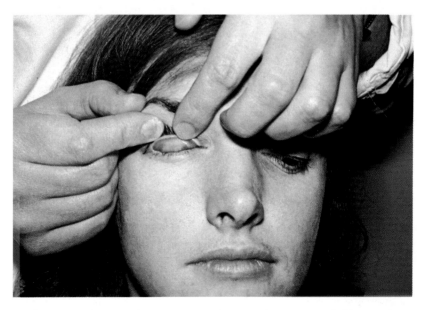

Fig. 9-3 On everting the upper lid, note any foreign body that is present. With magnification, one can view the upper margin of the tarsal plate and see pathologic changes. On reversing the procedure, pull the upper lid forward while the patient looks up.

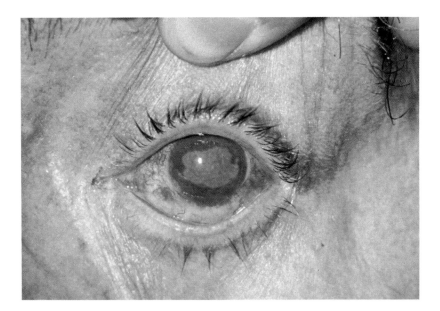

Fig. 9-4 If there is a loss of the corneal epithelium, then the fluoroscein dye will fluoresce as a bright green stain. This is particularly more noticeable if a cobalt blue filter is used. Filter paper impregnated with fluoroscein is available. The dry form of fluoroscein does not carry the risk of contamination. Fluoroscein strips may be placed in the outer or inferior fornix of the eye. The drop may be applied to the fluoroscein strip or the natural tears may wet the fluoroscein strip.

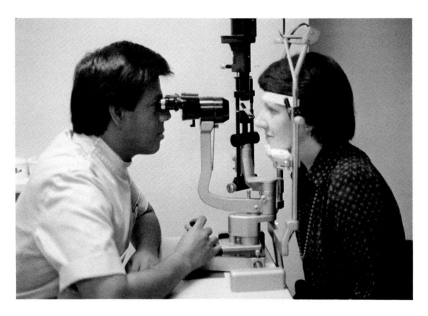

Fig. 9-5 The slitlamp microscope is capable of examining the anterior half of the eye under magnification. This is essentially a microscope of low power that can provide a slit, thin beam of light to provide an optical section of the cornea and lens as well as viewing the iris.

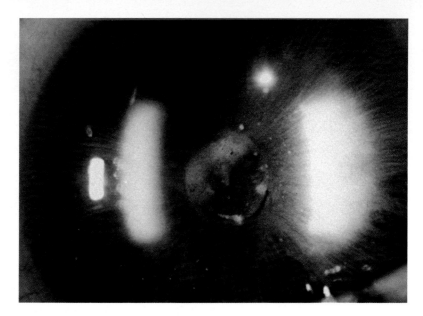

Fig. 9-6 The curved beam of light that strikes the cornea passes onward over the anterior chamber of the eye and then strikes the iris. In this view, the anterior chamber has some white spots that are aggregates of cells that denote an inflammatory pathologic condition inside the eye. The lens itself has many precipitates on the front surface and also has adhesions of the iris because of the lens surface.

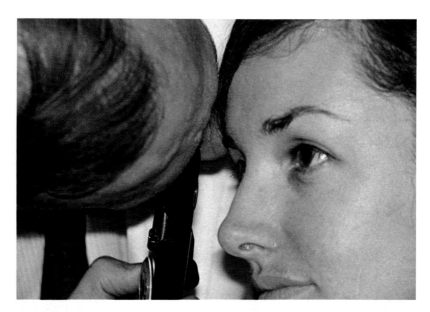

Fig. 9-7 The examiner starts about 10 inches in front of the eye and with high plus-power examines the external portion of the eye from afar. He or she then gets as close as possible turning the dial on the ophthalmoscope towards zero. The examiner should use his or her right eye with the ophthalmoscope in the right hand when looking at the right eye of the patient. This should be reversed when examining the left eye. The head should be firmly against a head rest if possible. Sitting positions are more desirable if standing positions lead to wobbling.

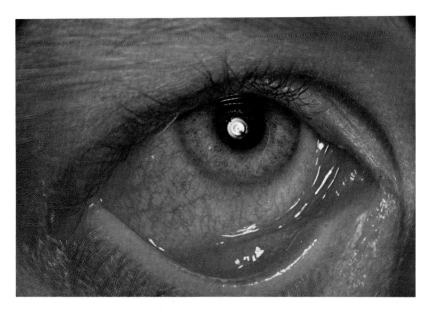

Fig. 9-8   The cornea and iris remain clear but there is extensive redness on the white bulbar conjunctiva and in the fornix and the pupil conjunctiva of the lower eyelid. This is a classic case of conjunctivitis. There is less redness toward the limbus than toward the conjunctiva. Conjunctivitis is an acute inflammatory condition that is usually viral or bacterial in nature. Classic symptoms of soreness, grittiness, and a red, congested eye are typical. It may be monocular or bilateral.

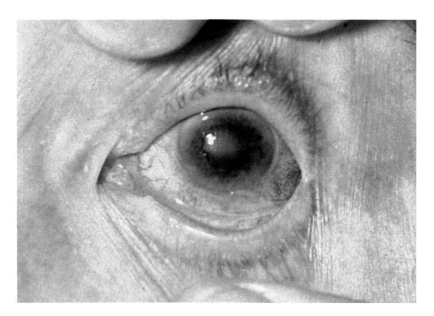

Fig. 9-9   This is a case of acute glaucoma. There is corneal haze with a dilated fixed pupil. Haze is the result of corneal edema. Increased pressure will be found on tonometry.

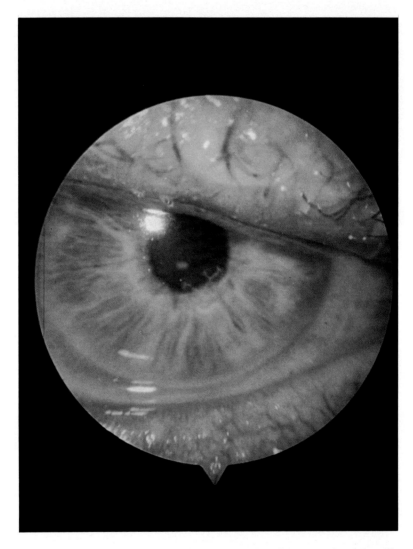

Fig. 9-10 Instillation of fluoroscein reveals a dendritic pattern of green on the cornea. The patient may or may not complain of soreness and blurring of vision. The fluoroscein stain and pattern of the corneal defect is *pathonomonic* of the dendritic ulcer.

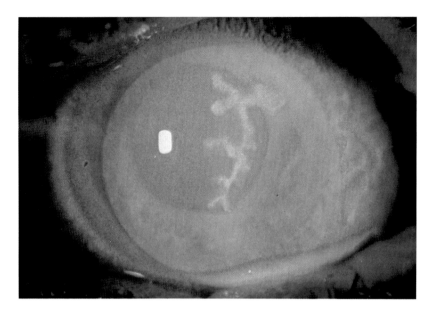

Fig. 9-11 The fluoroscein can be made more obvious by using a cobalt blue light with the slitlamp microscope.

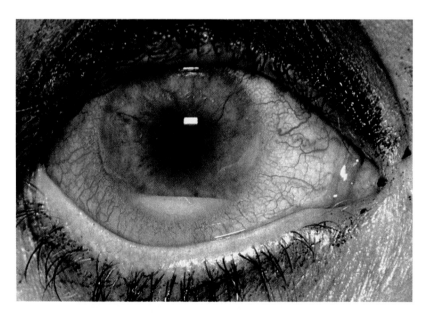

Fig. 9-12 Hypopyon. The eye is congested and there is a white level of material in the lower portion of the anterior chamber. This is a reaction to organisms that are within the interior of the eye. It is a danger sign. It is also dangerous to prescribe local steroids at this stage. The purulent material may lead to a panophthalmitis and should be referred urgently to a specialist.

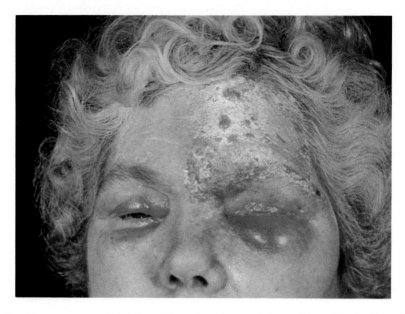

Fig. 9-13 Herpes zoster ophthalmicus. Edema in and around the eyelid combined with vesicles in any branches of the fifth or trigeminal nerve associated with pain is indicative of this picture. Sometimes in the early stages only a few vesicles may be present.

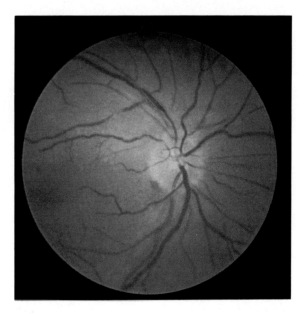

Fig. 9-14 Hypertensive retinopathy. There is a narrowing of the caliber of the arterioles and crossing of these arteriole over the veins, and a few hemorrhages may be seen.

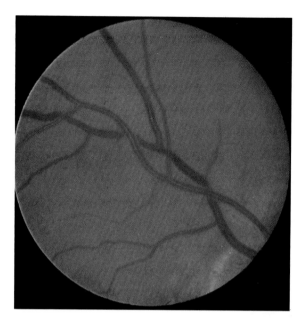

Fig. 9-15 Arterial changes show a silver wire reflection from the arteries with marked arteriovenous nipping.

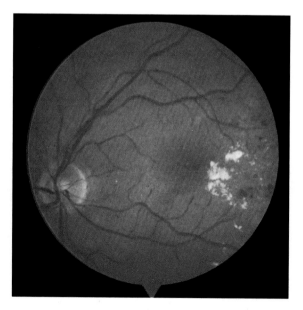

Fig. 9-16 Diabetic retinopathy. The retinal changes are predominantly at the posterior pole with microaneurysms and "dot and blot" hemorrhages, together with hard exudates in the macular area.

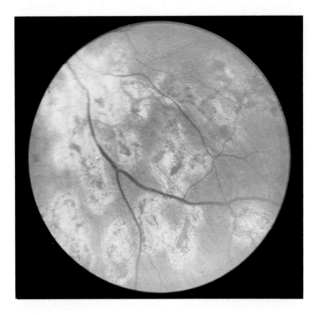

Fig. 9-17   Separate burns of the retina after light coagulation by laser. This was a treatment for a diabetic patient in which neovascularization was found in the deep bed.

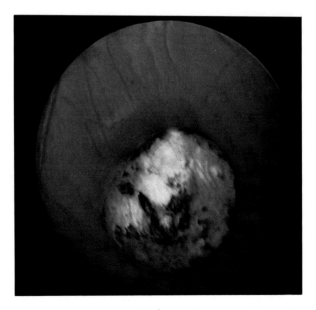

Fig. 9-18   Toxoplasmosis choroidoretinitis. There is a large active focus with scarring and black proliferation of pigment.

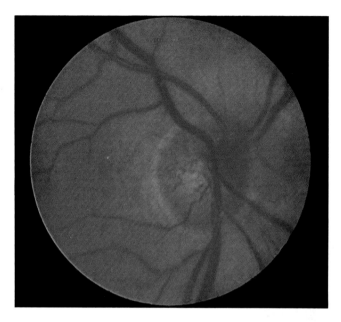

Fig. 9-19 Papilledema. There is a congestion of the disc with fine capillaries, particularly on the nasal side. There is an absence of venous pulsation and early swelling of the disc margin.

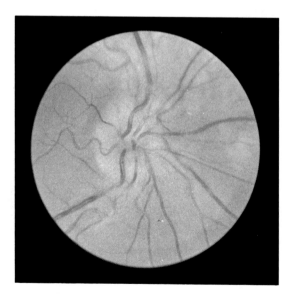

Fig. 9-20 A further stage of papilledema. There is gross swelling of the disc. Edema may be seen by partial transillumination of the disc margin.

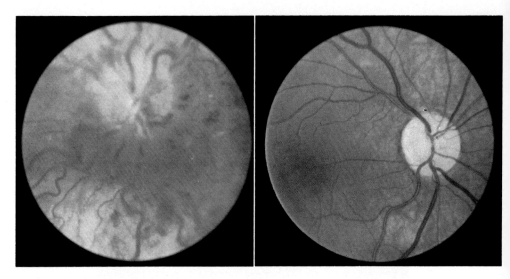

Fig. 9-21   A severe form of papilledema. The disc margins are completely obliterated and there is gross swelling with multiple hemorrhages.

Fig. 9-22   Optic atrophy. The disc is pale.

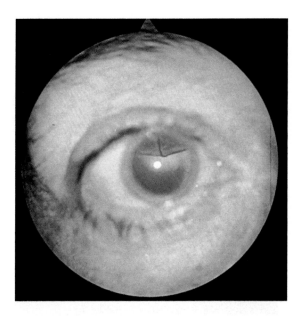

Fig. 9-23   Retinal detachment. The patient noted a clouding of the inferior portion of her vision. This corresponds with the retina, which is separating at the top of the globe. It is uncommon to see the retina as noted in this picture. Treatment is urgently required before the macula detaches.

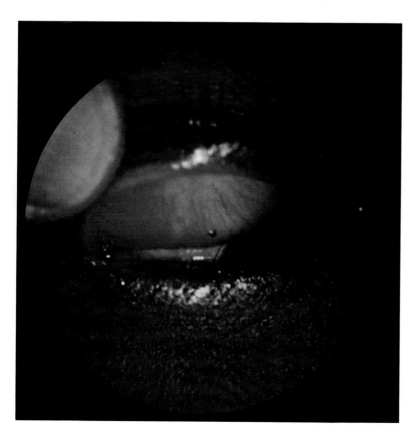

Fig. 9-24 Foreign body under the eyelid. The lid is everted and the foreign body lies against the upper tarsal margin of the conjunctiva. This should be removed with a Q-tip.

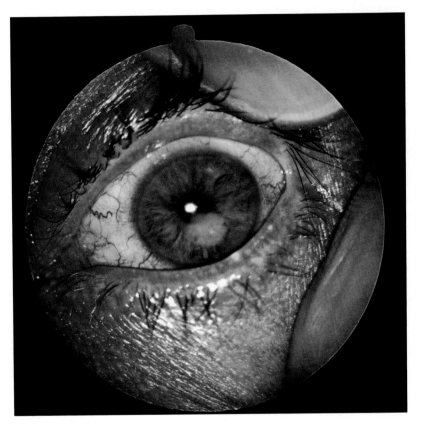

Fig. 9-25 Traumatic corneal erosion. The patient was injured with a fingernail and denuded the epithelium.

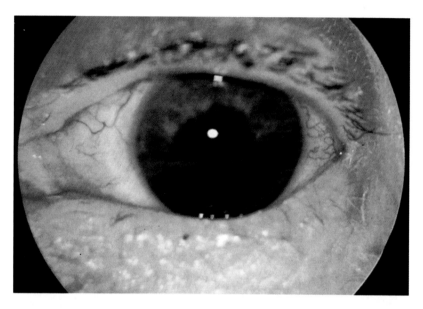

Fig. 9-26   Hyphema. The lower half of the eye is filled with a darkening blood. The blood is usually bright and clear initially and gradually becomes dark. The represents a serious contusion of the globe.

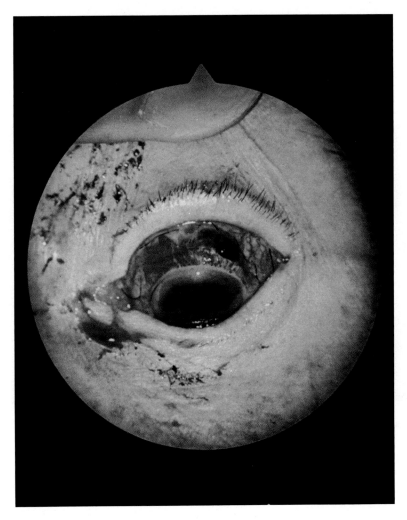

Fig. 9-27   Rupture of the globe. A blow has split the coats of the eye concentrically with the limbus with rupture of the choroid through the sclera.

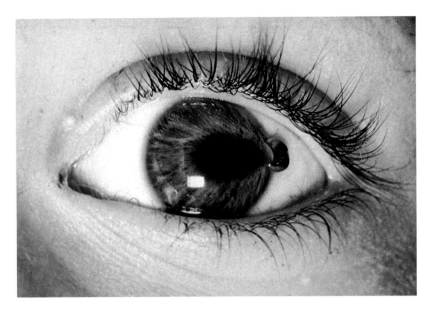

Fig. 9-28 Penetrating eye injury. While the patient was using a hammer and chisel on concrete, a piece of concrete chipped off and flew into the eye. The iris has prolapsed at the limbal margin and there is distortion of the pupil. This is an emergency for immediate admission and suturing.

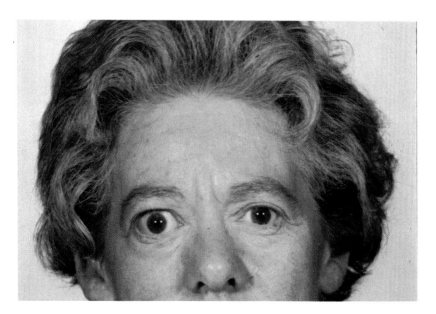

Fig. 9-29 Proptosis and lid retraction on the patient's right side. The eye is being pushed forward. A tumor or thyroid condition must be differentiated.

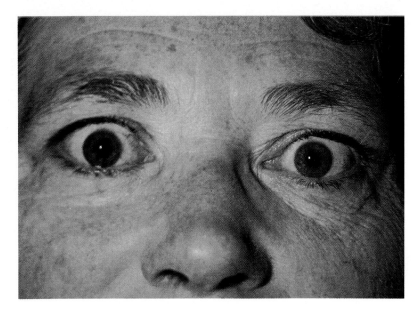

Fig. 9-30 Thyrotoxicosis, with bilateral, symmetrical lid retraction with sclera showing above the iris.

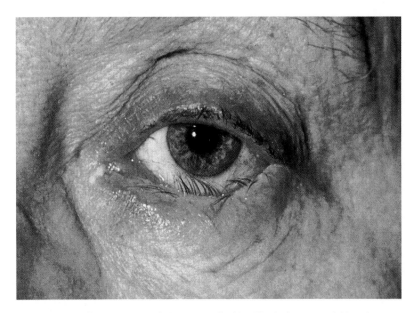

Fig. 9-31 Entropion. The eyelid and lashes are rolled in. The lashes are rubbing the cornea, particularly when the patient looks down.

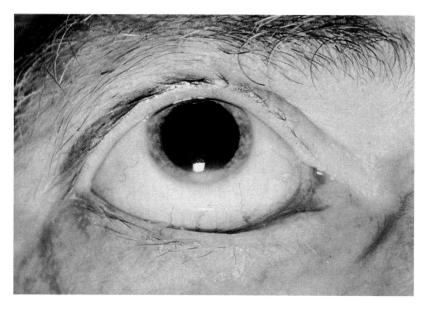

Fig. 9-32 Ectropion. In older people the lower lid loses its tone and drops away from the globe, particularly on the medial side. This can result in tearing as a result of the abnormal lid position.

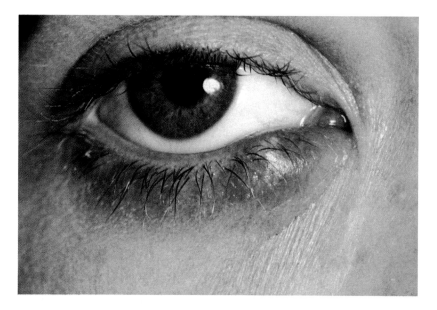

Fig. 9-33 Stye or acute hordeolum. This is an acute infective process involving the lash follicles.

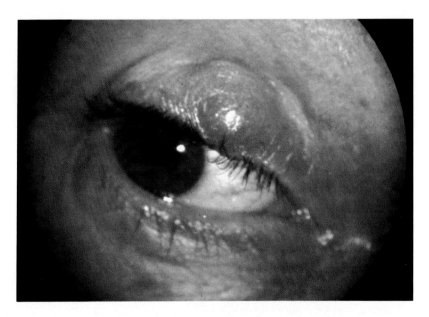

Fig. 9-34 Meibomian cyst. A swelling of the meibomian glands. This is a granuloma from eruption of sebum outside the walls of the gland.

Appendixes

Appendix A
Ocular Complications of Systemic Diseases

Disease	Possible ocular findings
Diabetes mellitus	• Background retinopathy: retinal hemorrhages, exudates, microaneurysms • Preproliferative retinopathy: cotton-wool spots, intraretinal microvascular abnormalities • Proliferative retinopathy: neovascularization, preretinal hemorrhage, vitreous hemorrhage, retinal detachment
Graves' disease	Lid retraction, exposure keratopathy, chemosis and injection, restriction of eye movements, proptosis, compressive optic neuropathy
Hypertension	Sclerosis of vessels in longstanding disease; narrowing of vessels, retinal hemorrhages, and/or exudates in severe hypertension
Rheumatoid arthritis and other collagen vascular diseases	Dry eye, episcleritis, scleritis, peripheral corneal ulceration and/or melting
Cancer	Metastatic disease to choroid may result in retinal detachment; disease in the orbit can result in proptosis and restriction of eye movements (for example, breast or lung cancer)

Appendix B
Lifesaving Ocular Signs

Findings	Clinical significance
White pupil	In an infant, retinoblastoma must be ruled out.
Aniridia (iris appears absent)	May be autosomal dominant (2/3s) or sporadic inheritance. In sporadic cases where the short arm of chromosome 11 is deleted, there is a 90% risk of developing Wilms' tumor; the risk in other sporadic cases is approximately 20%.
Thickened corneal nerves (slitlamp)	Part of the multiple endocrine neoplasia syndrome type IIB. Must rule out medullary carcinoma of the thyroid, pheochromocytoma, and parathyroid adenomas.
Retinal angioma	May be part of the Von Hippel-Lindau syndrome. Autosomal dominant inheritance with variable penetrance. Must rule out hemangioblastomas of the central nervous system, renal cell carcinoma, and pheochromocytoma.
Multiple pigmented patches of fundus	Lesions represent patches of congenital hypertrophy of the retinal pigment epithelium. May be part of Gardner's syndrome characterized by multiple premalignant intestinal polyps together with benign soft tissue tumors (lipomas, fibromas, sebaceous cysts) and osteomas of the skull and jaw. A complete gastrointestinal investigation is indicated. If Gardner's syndrome is diagnosed, prophylactic colectomy is indicated because of the potential for malignant degeneration of colonic polyps.
Third nerve palsy with a dilated pupil	Must rule out an intracranial aneurysm or neoplastic lesion. CT scan should be performed on an emergency basis.
Papilledema	Must rule out an intracranial mass lesion. CT scan should be performed on an emergency basis.
Pigmentary degeneration of the retina and motility disturbance	May represent the Kearns-Sayre syndrome. Must rule out a cardiac conduction defect diturbance with an annual electrocardiogram. May develop an intraventricular conduction defect, bundle block, bifascicular disease, or complete heart block. Patient must be prepared for the possible need to implant a pacemaker.

Appendix C
Ocular Complications of Systemic Medications

Medication	Ocular complications
Amiodarone	Superficial keratopathy
Chlorpromazine	Anterior subcapsular cataracts
Corticosteroids	Posterior subcapsular cataracts, glaucoma
Digitalis	Blurred vision, disturbed color vision
Ethambutol	Optic neuropathy
Indomethacin	Superficial keratopathy
Isoniazid	Optic neuropathy
Nalidixic acid	Papilledema
Hydroxychloroquine	Superficial keratopathy and bull's-eye maculopathy
Tetracycline	Papilledema
Thioridazine	Pigmentary degeneration of the retina
Vitamin A	Papilledema

Appendix D
I. Differential Diagnosis of the Nontraumatic Red Eye

	Condition		
Feature	Acute conjunctivitis	Acute iritis	Acute glaucoma
Symptoms	Redness, tearing +/− discharge	Redness, pain photophobia	Redness, severe pain, nausea, vomiting
Appearance	Conjunctival injection	Ciliary injection	Diffuse injection
Vision	Normal, can be blurred secondary to discharge	Moderate reduction	Marked reduction, halo vision
Cornea	Clear	May see keratic precipitates	Hazy secondary to edema
Pupil	Normal	Small, sluggish to light	Semidilated, nonreactive
Secretions	Tearing to purulent	Tearing	Tearing
Test and comments	Smears may show cause: bacterial infection = polycytes, bacteria; viral infection = monocytes; allergy = eosinophils	Slitlamp will show cells and flare in the anterior chamber	Elevated intraocular pressure
Treatment	Antibiotic	Steroids, cycloplegics	Pilocarpine, Betagan Diamox, mannitol, laser surgery

2. Differential Diagnosis of Viral, Bacterial, and Allergic Conjunctivitis

Feature	Viral	Bacterial	Allergy
Discharge	Watery	Purulent	Watery
Itching	Minimal	Minimal	Marked
Preauricular lymph node	Common	Absent	Absent
Stain and smear	Monocytes Lymphocytes	Bacteria Polycytes	Eosinophils

Appendix E
Differential Diagnosis of the Red Eye in Contact Lens Wearers

Diagnosis	Findings	Mechanism	Treatment
Corneal abrasion	Epithelial defect Stains with fluorescein.	Mechanical Hypoxia.	Antibiotic drops (such as tobramycin)
Superficial punctate keratitis	Punctate corneal staining	Mechanical. Chemical toxicity	Artificial tears (such as Refresh ocular lubricant)
Giant papillary conjunctivitis	Papillary reaction of superior tarsal conjunctiva	Immunologic. Mechanical	Mast cell stabilizer (such as Vlstacrom drops)
Sterile infiltrates	Corneal infiltrate. Epithelium usually intact	Immunologic	Antibiotic drops (assume infected)
Infected ulcer	Corneal infiltrate with ulceration. Stains with fluorescein	Infection, (for example, *Pseudomomas, Staphylococcus aureus*)	Corneal scraping for Gram stain and culture. Fortified antibiotic drops

Appendix F Estimating Visual Loss

LOSS OF CENTRAL VISION IN ONE EYE

Visual acuity for distance (Snellen	Snellen	Meters (D)	Jaeger	Percent visual efficiency*
20/20	14/14	0.35	1−	100
20/25	14/18	0.44	2−	96
20/30	14/21	0.59	—	91
20/40	14/28	0.71	3	84
20/50	14/35	0.88	6	77
20/60	14/42	1.08	—	70
20/70	14/49	1.30	7	64
20/80	14/56	—	8	59
20/100	14/70	1.76	11−	49
20/160	14/112	—	14−	29
20/200	14/140	3.53	—	20
20/400	14/280	7.06	—	3

*The percentage of visual efficiency of the two eyes may be determined by the following formula:

$$\frac{(3 \times \%\text{Visual efficiency of better eye}) + \%\text{Visual efficiency of poorer eye}}{4} = \%\text{Binocular visual effiency}$$

ESTIMATING LOSS OF VISUAL FIELD

A visual field test is performed on the perimeter with a 3 mm test object in each of the eight 45-degree meridians. The sum of each of these meridians is added and the percentage of visual meridians is added and the percentage of visual efficiency arrived at by dividing by 485, the total of a normal field. For example:

Normal field	Degrees
Temporally	85
Down and temporally	85
Down	55
Nasally	55
Up and nasally	55
Down and nasally	50
Up	45
Up and temporally	55
TOTAL	485

Constricted field	Degrees
Temporally	45
Down and temporally	25
Down	30
Down and nasally	25
Nasally	25
Up and nasally	25
Up	25
Up and temporally	35
TOTAL	235

$$\%\text{Visual efficiency}\ \frac{235 \times 100}{485} = 46\%$$

Appendix G Short Forms in Clinical Use

Acc   accommodation
add   addition
od   right eye *(oculus dexter)*
os   left eye *(oculus sinister)*
ou   both eyes *(oculi unitas)*
RE   right eye
LE   left eye
NV   near vision
PH   pinhole
V   vision or visual acuity
mm   millimeter
mg   milligram
SC   without correction
CC   with correction
HM   hand movements
LP   light perception
MR   Maddox rod
L & A   light and accommodation
EOMB   extraocular muscle balance
EOM   extraocular movements
CF   counting fingers
XP   exophoria
XT   exotropia
W   wearing
IOP   intraocular pressure
T   tension
ung   ointment
A   applanation tensions
KP   keratic precipitates
PSC   posterior subcapsular cataract
ASC   anterior subcapsular cataract
ET   esotropia
°   degree
Δ   prism diopter

D   diopter
RH   right hyperphoria
LH   left hyperphoria
PD or IPD   interpupillary distance
NPA   near point of accommodation
NPC   near point of convergence
MR   medial rectus (muscle)
LR   lateral rectus (muscle)
SR   superior rectus (muscle)
IR   inferior rectus (muscle)
SO   superior oblique (muscle)
IO   inferior oblique (muscle)
BO   base out
BI   base in
BD   base down
BU   base up
NRC   normal retinal correspondence
ARC   abnormal retinal correspondence
J1, J2, J3, etc.   test types for reading vision
N5, N6, etc.   test types for near vision
bid or bd   twice daily
tid or td   three times daily
qid   four times daily
ac   before meals
pc   after meals
ic   between meals
ne rep or non rep   do not repeat
oculent   eye ointment
per os or po   orally, by mouth
prn   when required, as necessary
qh   every hour
q2h   every 2 hours
qs   quantity sufficient
stat   at once

The following abbreviations may sometimes be found on ophthalmic charts:

VA   visual acuity
VAc or VAcc   visual acuity with correction
VAs or VAsc   visual acuity without correction
VA   visual acuity with the unaided
OT   eye
AT or Appl   ocular tension
ST   applanation tension
EOM   Schiøtz tension extraocular muscle
E₁   esophoria for distance

E'   esophoria for near
ET₁   esotropia for distance
ET'   esotropia for near
X₁   exophoria for distance
X'   exophoria for near
E(T)   intermittent esotropia
X(T)   intermittent exotropia
dd   disc diameters

Appendix H Vision and Driving

Good vision is essential for the proper and safe operation of a motor vehicle. Generally available vision-testing instruments can be used to ascertain if an individual has adequate vision to meet specific standards set by the various state licensing jurisdictions. Because of the increasing injury and death toll resulting from traffic crashes, many of which may be related to visual impairment, physicians should consider it a medical obligation to diagnose visual deficiencies and to inform the patient of potential hazards involved in driving with such deficiencies.

There is no practical way of testing alertness or cerebral perception of what the eye focuses on, but it is important for drivers to have their eyes periodically examined for defects that can be evaluated. This is particularly important for those drivers with significant progressive visual deterioration.

In general, if any doubt exists about an individual's visual ability to operate an automobile safely, the physician should not hesitate to recommend road tests for specific evaluation of visual skills.

Visual acuity. Automobile drivers with corrected central visual acuity of 20/40 or better generally read traffic signs and note obstructions, vehicles, and pedestrians while driving at usual speeds, whereas those with optimally corrected vision of 20/70 or less in the better eye have a serious limitation and should not drive.

Drivers with visual acuity between 20/40 and 20/70 should be referred to an ophthalmologist to ascertain if their vision can be improved. The physician, in serving the best interests of patients, should consider the conditions under which each patient drives and the presence or absence of associated defects. The physician is then in a position to advise the patient against driving under certain conditions, such as congested traffic, hazardous road conditions, bad weather, high speed, or at night. It is hoped that continuing research will more exactly define the criteria on which to advise patients.

One-eyed drivers and spectacle-corrected aphakic drivers have visual field limitations and present an increased risk of intersectional crashes. Most postoperative aphakic patients, particularly those in advanced years, also have increased difficulty with night vision and dynamic visual responses. They require special evaluation. Preoperative cataract patients with early to moderate changes in the lenses of the eye similarly have night-driving limitations (glare intolerance and reduced night vision) that generally preclude night driving. Patients requiring pupil-constricting medication, as in the control of chronic glaucoma, also have limitation for night operation.

Visual fields. Visual fields are obviously important for safe driving, since a driver must possess some breadth or lateral awareness to pass approaching vehicles safely and to be aware of vehicles or pedestrians approaching from the side.

Although visual form fields of 140 degrees generally are considered adequate for drivers of private motor vehicles, that figure should be considered as the absolute minimum for drivers of commercial and passenger-carrying vehicles. Such drivers also must have coordinate use of both eyes, as well as a corrected acuity of at least 20/30 in the better eye and no worse than 20/40 in the poorer eye. Individuals with lesser fields have driver limitation and must be evaluated for the driving of private vehicles on the basis of the conditions under which they drive, the amount of lateral vision retained, and underlying ocular pathologic condition.

Individuals with markedly constricted fields, such as those from advanced glaucoma or retinitis pigmentosa, have distinct driver limitation and should be so advised.

Ocular muscle imbalance. Ocular muscle imbalance (heterophoria) is an indirect cause of automotive crashes in that it may cause driver fatigue. If sudden diplopia occurs, the crash may be directly attributable to the diplopia. Therefore, patients with uncontrolled or intermittent diplopia have definite driver limitation.

Color blindness. Impaired or defective color vision has been considered a potential cause of highway accidents. However, most traffic lights have been standardized, at least regionally, and it is doubtful that this deficiency is too hazardous, except in severe cases. A completely color-blind, or achromatic, individual has very poor vision and should not drive under any circumstance. This also applies to the very limited number of individuals who have severe protanopia, or red deficiency.

Dark adaptation. Dark adaptation and susceptibility to glare are of great importance in night driving, but testing procedures and standards are still largely empiric and not a component of routine eye tests. Dark glasses should never be worn for night driving, and the windshield tinting should be limited to the upper one third.

Depth perception. Current testing techniques in the near range do not have significant correlation with distance visual requirements in driving but are adequate for determining visual ability for such tasks as parking. The road test, however, is still the best and most practical guide in this area.

Appendix I Metric Conversion

	When you know	Multiply by	To find
LENGTH	inches (in)	2.5	centimeters (cm)
	feet (ft)	30.4	centimeters
	miles (mi)	1.6	kilometers (km)
AREA	square inches (in²)	6.5	square centimeters (cm²)
	square miles (mi²)	2.6	square kilometers (im²)
WEIGHT	ounces (oz)	28.3	grams (g)
	pounds (lb)	0.45	kilograms (kg)
VOLUME AND CAPACITY	teaspoons (tsp)	4.6	milliliters (ml)
	tablespoons (Tbsp)	14.0	milliliters
	fluid ounces (fl oz)	28.0	milliliters
	cups (C)	0.227	liters (L)
	pints (pt)	0.568	liters
	quarts (qt)	1.1	liters
	gallons (gal)	4.5	liters
	cubic inches (cu in)	16.3872	cubic centimeters (cc)
SPEED AND VELOCITY	miles per hour (mph)	1.609	kilometers per hour (km/h)
	feet per seconds (fps)	30.4	centimeters per second (cm/s)
TEMPERATURE	Fahrenheit temperature (°F)	5/9 (after subtracting 32)	Celsius temperature (°C)

MASS

1 lb = 0.454 kg
1 kg = 2.205 lb
½ oz = 14.17 g
1 oz = 28.35 g

LENGTH

1 in = 2.540 cm
1 ft = 0.3048 m
1 mi = 1.609 km
10 millimeters (mm) = 1 cm = 0.3937 in
100 cm = 1 m = 39.37 in
1000 m = 1 km = 0.62137 mi

VOLUME

1 q = 1.1366 L
1 gal = 4.4561 L
½ oz = 15 ml
1 oz = 30 ml
10 ml = 1 cc = 0.338 fl oz
10 cl = 1 deciliter (dl) = 6.1025 in²
10 dl = 1 L = 1.0567 liquid qt
100 L = 1 hectoliter (hl) = 26.418 gal

TEMPERATURE

0° Celsius = 32° Fahrenheit
0° Fahrenheit = >17.8° Celsius
100° Celsium = 212° Fahrenheit

Appendix J Translations of Commonly Asked Questions and Commands

English	French
HISTORY	

English	French
1. What is your name?	1. Quel est votre nom?
2. What is your address?	2. Quelle est votre addresse?
3. When were you born?	3. Quel est votre jour de naissance?
4. What trouble are you having with your eyes?	4. Quel problème avez-vous avec les yeux?
5. Are you having pain?	5. Ça fait mal?
6. Do your eyes itch?	6. Ça pique?
7. Have you had an eye injury?	7. Est-ce que les yeux ont été blessés?
8. Have you had an eye operation?	8. Est-ce que les yeux ont été opérés?
9. Did you get anything in your eye?	9. Y-a-t-il quelque chose dans les yeux?
10. Are you taking any eye drops?	10. Employez-vous des gouttes pour les yeux?
11. Do you have headaches?	11. Avez-vous des maux de têtes?
12. Do you wear glasses?	12. Portez-vous des lunettes?
13. How old are your glasses?	13. Et depuis quand?
14. Do you have trouble reading?	14. Pouvez-vous lire sans difficulté?
15. Do you see double?	15. Voyez-vous double?
16. Do you take pills?	16. Prenez-vous des médicaments?
For: heart	Pour: le coeur
diabetes	le diabète
blood pressure	la tension artérielle
17. Do you have any allergies?	17. Avez-vous des allergies?
To medicine	Aux médicaments?
Others	Ou à des autres choses?
18. Is there a history of diabetes or glaucoma in your family?	18. Y'a-t-ile diabète ou le glaucome dans votre famille?
19. Is there a history of eye problems?	19. Y'a-t-il des problèmes avec les yeux?

English	French
EXAMINATION	

English	French
20. Look straight.	20. Regardez tout droit.
21. Follow my light.	21. Suivez ma lumière.
22. Follow my finger.	22. Suivez mon doigt.
23. Can you count my fingers?	23. Pouvez-vous compter mes doigts?
24. Can you see my hand move?	24. Pouvez-vous voir bouger ma main?
25. Open your eyes. Close your eyes.	25. Ouvrez les yeux. Fermez les yeux.
26. Look at me.	26. Regardez-moi.
27. Is it clear?	27. Est-il clair?
28. Read this.	28. Lizes ça.
29. Which is better, one or two?	29. Le quel est mieux, un ou deux?

Translations of Commonly Asked Questions and Commands—cont'd

English	German

HISTORY

English	German
1. What is your name?	1. Ihr Name, bitte?
2. What is your address?	2. Ihre Anschrift, bitte?
3. When were you born?	3. Ihr Geburtsdatum, bitte?
4. What trouble are you having with your eyes?	4. Was für ein Problem haben Sie mit den Augen?
5. Are you having pain?	5. Haben Sie Schmerzen?
6. Do your eyes itch?	6. Tun Ihre Augen jucken?
7. Have you had any eye injury?	7. Haben Sie mal eine Augenverletzung gehabt?
8. Have you had an eye operation?	8. Haben Sie mal eine Augenoperation gehabt?
9. Did you get anything in your eye?	9. Ist irgendwas in Ihre Augen geraten?
10. Are you taking any eye drops?	10. Benützen Sie Augentropfen?
11. Do you have headaches?	11. Haben Sie Kopfschmerzen?
12. Do you wear glasses?	12. Tragen Sie Brillen?
13. How old are your glasses?	13. Seit wann tragen Sie Brillen?
14. Do you have trouble reading?	14. Haben Sie Schwierigkeiten beim Lesen?
15. Do you see double?	15. Sehen Sie doppelt?
16. Do you take pills?	16. Nämen Sie Pillen ein?
For: heart	Für Herz?
diabetes	Zuckerkrankheit
blood pressure	Blutdruck?
17. Do you have any allergies?	17. Haben Sie irgend Allergien?
To medicine	Gegen Medizin?
Others	Andere Allergien?
18. Is there a history of diabetes or glaucoma in your family?	18. Laufen Zuckerkrankheit oder Glaucom in Ihre Familie?
19. Is there a history of eye problems?	19. Laufen Augenkrankheit in Ihre Familie?

EXAMINATION

English	German
20. Look straight.	20. Schauen Sie gerade aus.
21. Follow my light.	21. Folgen Sie dem Licht.
22. Follow my finger.	22. Folgen Sie meinem Finger.
23. Can you count my fingers?	23. Zählen Sie meine Finger.
24. Can you see my hand move?	24. Können Sie Bewegung meiner Hand sehen?
25. Open your eyes. Close your eyes.	25. Öffnen Sie die Augen. Schliessen Sie die Augen.
26. Look at me.	26. Schauen Sie mich an.
27. Is it clear?	27. Erscheine ich klar?
28. Read this.	28. Lesen Sie dieses.
29. Which is better, one or two?	29. Was ist besser, eins oder zwei?

Translations of Commonly Asked Questions and Commands—cont'd

English	**Italian**

HISTORY

1. What is your name?	1. Come ti chiami?
2. What is your address?	2. Il tuo indirizzo.
3. When were you born?	3. La tua data di nascita.
4. What trouble are you having with your eyes?	4. Hai qualche problema con i tuoi occhi?
5. Are you having pain?	5. Senti dolore?
6. Do your eyes itch?	6. I tuoi occhi bruciano?
7. Have you had any eye injury?	7. Hai avuto un incidente agli occhi?
8. Have you had an eye operation?	8. Hai mai avuto una operazione agli occhi?
9. Did you get anything in your eye?	9. Cosa e' entrato nel tuo occhio?
10. Are you taking any eye drops?	10. Usi gocce per occhi?
11. Do you have headaches?	11. Hai dolori di testa?
12. Do you wear glasses?	12. Usi occhiali?
13. How old are your glasses?	13. Da quanto tempo usi questi occhiali?
14. Do you have trouble reading?	14. Riesci a leggere?
15. Do you see double?	15. Vedi doppio?
16. Do you take pills?	16. Usi pillole?
For: heart	Per: il cuore
diabetes	il diabete
blood pressure	la pressione
17. Do you have any allergies?	17. Hai allergie?
To medicine	a medicine
Others	di qualsiasi tipo
18. Is there a history of diabetes or glaucoma in your family?	18. C'e' qualche caso di diabete o glaucoma nella tua famiglia?
19. Is there a history of eye problems?	19. Qualcuno in famiglia ha avuto disturbi alla vista?

EXAMINATION

20. Look straight.	20. Guarda diritto.
21. Follow my light.	21. Segui la luce.
22. Follow my finger.	22. Segui il mio dito.
23. Can you count my fingers?	23. Quante dita vedi?
24. Can you see my hand move?	24. Vedi la mia mano muoversi?
25. Open your eyes. Close your eyes.	25. Apri gli occhi. Chiudi gli occhi.
26. Look at me.	26. Guardami.
27. Is it clear?	27. Vedi chiaro?
28. Read this.	28. Leggi.
29. Which is better, one or two?	29. Qual e' meglio, uno o due?

Translations of Commonly Asked Questions and Commands—cont'd

English	Polish

HISTORY

1. What is your name?
2. What is your address?
3. When were your born?
4. What trouble are you having with your eyes?
5. Are you having pain?
6. Do your eyes itch?
7. Have you had any eye injury?
8. Have you had an eye operation?
9. Did you get anything in your eye?
10. Are you taking any eye drops?
11. Do you have headaches?
12. Do you wear glasses?
13. How old are your glasses?
14. Do you have trouble reading?
15. Do you see double?
16. Do you take pills?
    For: Heart
        Diabetes
        Blood pressure
17. Do you have any allergies?
    To medicine
    Others
18. Is there a history of diabetes or glaucoma in your family?
19. Is there a history of eye problems?

EXAMINATION

20. Look straight.
21. Follow my light.
22. Follow my finger.
23. Can you count my fingers?
24. Can you see my hand move?
25. Open your eyes. Close your eyes.
26. Look at me.
27. Is it clear?
28. Read this.
29. Which is better, one or two?

---

1. Jak się pan (pani) nazywa?
2. Jaki jest pana (pani) adres?
3. Kiedy się pan urodził (pani urodziła)?
4. Jaki pan (pani) ma problem z oczami?
5. Czy pan (pani) odczuwa ból?
6. Czy pana (pani) swędzą oczy?
7. Czy oko było skaleczone?
8. Czy miał pan (miała pani) operację na oczy?
9. Czy coś się dostało do oka?
10. Czy bierze pan (pani) krople do oczu?
11. Czy cierpi pan (pani) na bole glowy?
12. Czy nosi pan (pani) okulary?
13. Jak dawno nosi pan (pani) te okulary?
14. Czy ma pan (pani) problemy z czytaniem?
15. Czy widzi pan (pani) podwójnie?
16. Czy bierze pan (pani) pastylki?
    Na: Serce
        Cukrzyce
        Wysoki ciśnienie
17. Czy cierpi pan (pani) na alergie?
    Na lekarstwa
    Inne
18. Czy ktośz rodziny cierpi na cukrzyce lub jaskre?
19. Czy ktośz rodziny ma problemy z oczami?

20. Proszę patrzeć prosto.
21. Proszę wodzić wzrokiem za światlem.
22. Proszę wodzić wzrokiem za moim palcem.
23. Czy może pan (pani) policzyć moje palce?
24. Czy widzi pan (pani) jak rusza się moja ręja?
25. Proszę otworzyć oczy. Proszé zamknąć oczy.
26. Proszę spojrzeć na mnie.
27. Czy to jest dobrze widoczne?
28. Proszę to przeczytać.
29. Które jest lepsze, pierwsze czy drugie?

Translations of Commonly Asked Questions and Commands—cont'd

English	Spanish

HISTORY

	English		Spanish
1.	What is your name?	1.	Su nombre, por favor.
2.	What is your address?	2.	Su dirección, por favor.
3.	When were you born?	3.	Su fecha de nacimiento, por favor.
4.	What trouble are you having with your eyes?	4.	¿Tiene usted dificultades con la vista?
5.	Are you having pain?	5.	¿Le duelen los ojos?
6.	Do your eyes itch?	6.	¿Le pican los ojos?
7.	Have you had any eye injury?	7.	¿Han recibido daño en alguna forma sus ojos?
8.	Have you had an eye operation?	8.	¿Ha sufrido usted alguna operación en los ojos?
9.	Did you get anything in your eye?	9.	¿Tiene algo en el ojo?
10.	Are you taking any eye drops?	10.	¿Está usted usando gotas para los ojos?
11.	Do you have headaches	11.	¿Sufre usted de dolores de cabeza?
12.	Do you wear glasses?	12.	¿Usa usted espejuelos (gafas)?
13.	How old are your glasses?	13.	¿Cuántos años tienen sus gafas?
14.	Do you have trouble reading?	14.	¿Les molestan cuando lee?
15.	Do you see double?	15.	¿Ve doble?
16.	Do you take pills?	16.	¿Toma usted medicinas?
	For: heart		para: el corazón
	diabetes		la diabetes
	blood pressure		la presión arterial?
17.	Do you have any allergies?	17.	¿Es usted alérgico?
	To medicine		a las medicinas
	Others		a otras cosas?
18.	Is there a history of diabetes or glaucoma in your family?	18.	¿Existen o han existido casos de diabetes o de glaucoma en su familia?
19.	Is there a history of eye problems?	19.	¿Existen o han existido problemas de la vista en la familia?

EXAMINATION

	English		Spanish
20.	Look straight.	20.	¡Mire directamente hacia delante!
21.	Follow my light.	21.	¡Siga la luz con sus ojos!
22.	Follow my finger.	22.	¡Siga mi dedo con sus ojos!
23.	Can you count my fingers?	23.	¿Puede contar los dedos?
24.	Can you see my hand move?	24.	¿Ve mi mano cuando se mueve?
25.	Open your eyes. Close your eyes.	25.	¡Abra los ojos! ¡Cierre los ojos!
26.	Look at me.	26.	¡Míreme!
27.	Is it clear?	27.	¿Lo ve claramente?
28.	Read this.	28.	¡Lea esto!
29.	Which is better, one or two?	29.	¿De los dos cuál es el mejor, el uno o el dos?

Index

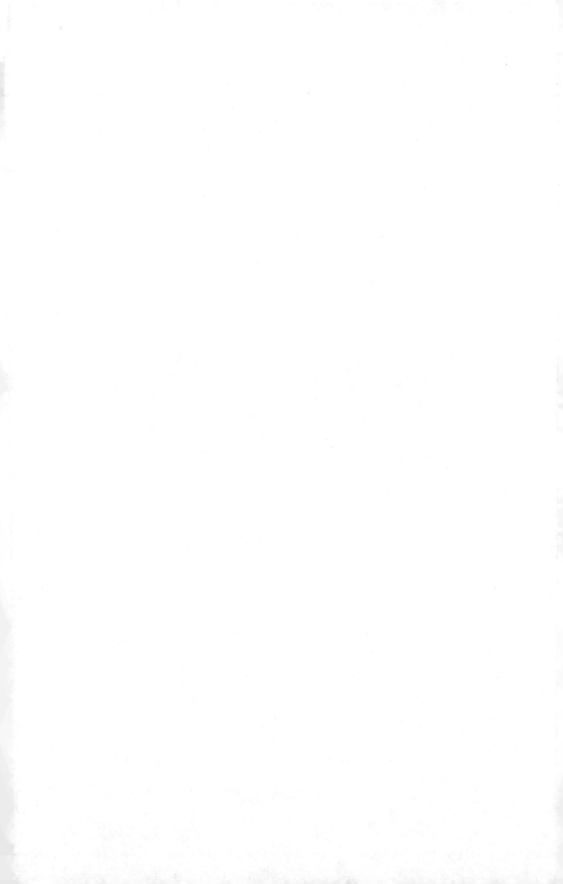